Handbook of Male Infertility and Andrology

Handbook of Male Infertility and Andrology

Naveenchandra Acharya
MS MNAMS DNB MRCS (UK) MCh (Uro) PGI (Chandi)
Consultant
Urologist, Andrologist and Microsurgeon
Specialist in Male Infertility and Impotence
Ramayya Pramila Urology and Laparoscopy Hospitals
Hyderabad, Telangana, India

Sharmila Majumdar
MS in Sexuality, PhD
Behavior Modification and Cognitive Restructuring
Ramayya Pramila Urology and Laparoscopy Hospitals
Hyderabad, Telangana, India

Ramesh Ramayya
FRCS (Eng) FRCS (Edin) ChM (Liverpool)
Consultant
Urologist and Endourologist
Specialist in HIFU and Laser Surgery
Chairman
Ramayya Pramila Urology and Laparoscopy Hospitals
Hyderabad, Telangana, India

Foreword
SK Singh

JAYPEE *The Health Sciences Publisher*
New Delhi | London | Philadelphia | Panama

Jaypee Brothers Medical Publishers (P) Ltd.

Headquarters
Jaypee Brothers Medical Publishers (P) Ltd.
4838/24, Ansari Road, Daryaganj
New Delhi 110 002, India
Phone: +91-11-43574357
Fax: +91-11-43574314
Email: jaypee@jaypeebrothers.com

Overseas Offices

J.P. Medical Ltd.
83, Victoria Street, London
SW1H 0HW (UK)
Phone: +44-20 3170 8910
Fax: +44(0) 20 3008 6180
E-mail: info@jpmedpub.com

Jaypee-Highlights Medical Publishers Inc.
City of Knowledge, Bld. 237, Clayton
Panama City, Panama
Phone: +1 507-301-0496
Fax: +1 507-301-0499
E-mail: cservice@jphmedical.com

Jaypee Medical Inc.
The Bourse
111, South Independence Mall East
Suite 835, Philadelphia, PA 19106, USA
Phone: +1 267-519-9789
E-mail: jpmed.us@gmail.com

Jaypee Brothers Medical Publishers (P) Ltd.
17/1-B, Babar Road, Block-B, Shaymali
Mohammadpur, Dhaka-1207
Bangladesh
Mobile: +08801912003485
E-mail: jaypeedhaka@gmail.com

Jaypee Brothers Medical Publishers (P) Ltd.
Bhotahity, Kathmandu, Nepal
Phone: +977-9741283608
E-mail: kathmandu@jaypeebrothers.com

Website: www.jaypeebrothers.com
Website: www.jaypeedigital.com

Inquiries for bulk sales may be solicited at: jaypee@jaypeebrothers.com

Handbook of Male Infertility and Andrology

First Edition : **2015**

ISBN: 978-93-5152-626-1

Printed at : Samrat Offset Pvt. Ltd.

Dedicated to

Almighty Sai

Foreword

It is with immense pleasure I am writing the foreword for this important book. Although andrology has been recognized as a subspecialty and special fellowship programs have been introduced in this field in Western countries; this field is yet to be established fully in many countries. With the evolution of Industries and Information Technology Sector; the lifestyle of the people also has changed. With the stress levels climbing up; more and more patients are facing health issues related to andrology. The expanding knowledge and awareness about sexual and fertility problems have also contributed to increasing number of patients with related ailments coming to the outpatient department of Urology. It is worth appreciating the efforts of three distinguished specialists who have brought this concise book to present an overview of this upcoming subspecialty. It is really praiseworthy. This will help aspiring andrologists to catch-up with the rapidly expanding field of andrology and percolate the knowledge to the needy.

This handbook has been written in a simple language and the authors have tried to cover a wide spectrum of areas in andrology. It will definitely be a good source of knowledge and reference for budding andrologists, postgraduates and also for the general physicians. The authors have contributed through their valuable clinical experience to make the book as a compendium in the field of andrology. It covers a vast area ranging from biological aspects of sexuality and fertility to the recent advances including robotics. What makes the book even more lucid is covering topics on female sexual dysfunction extensively and dedicating a chapter on "Setting up an Andrology Suite" which will be of great help to a clinician in establishing the clinic.

I wish this endeavor of the authors a grand success.

SK Singh
Professor, Department of Urology
Postgraduate Institute of Medical Education and Research (PGIMER)
Chandigarh, India

Preface

The book covers male infertility, erectile dysfunction and certain other andrological disorders such as priapism, penile fractures and Peyronie's disease. The initial chapter covers anatomical and physiological aspects of male reproductive system. One chapter has been written on male menopause—its diagnosis and management. The medical and surgical management of the above disorders are covered in the subsequent chapters.

The male infertility portion covers—management of oligospermia, varicocele, cryptorchidism and reconstructive andrological procedures. The ever-neglected subject of female sexual dysfunction has been covered extensively in a separate chapter. A special chapter has been dedicated to vasectomy—its evolution and newer forms of vasectomy such as non-scalpel and non-needle vasectomies and complications and a special mention regarding its reversal.

The pharmacotherapy in andrology has been covered separately for the summarization of the medical management of the common andrological conditions. For budding andrologists, a chapter has been dedicated to setting up andrology suite. The latest innovations such as robotic microsurgical procedures have been included in the last chapter to apprise the postgraduate students about the new technologies developing in this field.

We hope that this book will be of value for general practitioners, urologists and budding andrologists.

Naveenchandra Acharya
Sharmila Majumdar
Ramesh Ramayya

Acknowledgments

We would like to express gratitude to all the patients without whom the book could not have been published. We thank and gratefully acknowledge Dr GP Ramayya and Smt Pramila Devi, the founders of the Ramayya Pramila Urology and Laparoscopy Hospitals, Hyderabad, Telangana, India. They were the visionaries who pioneered the concept of standalone urosurgical center which allowed us to work with pride in a state-of-the-art patient centric hospital.

We acknowledge and thank M/s Jaypee Brothers Medical Publishers (P) Ltd., New Delhi, India, for giving us a platform to publish our views and experience regarding male infertility and andrology.

Contents

1. Anatomy and Physiology of the Male Reproductive System **1**

Male Reproductive System *1*
Anatomy of the Sperm *1*
Hormonal Considerations *2*
Testicular Anatomy *3*
Seminiferous Tubules *4*
Epididymis *4*
Male Erectile Apparatus *4*

2. Erectile Dysfunction **8**

Prevalence *8*
Pathophysiology *8*
Causes *8*
Evaluation *9*
Diagnosis *9*
Practical Tips *10*
Laboratory Tests *10*
Other Tests *10*
Treatment *13*

3. Intracavernosal Injection **16**

Intracavernosal Injection of Vasoactive Drugs—Practical Approach *16*
Drugs and Pathophysiology *16*
Pathophysiology *17*
Home Administered Injection *17*
Patient Acceptance and Drop-Out *18*
Serious Adverse Effects *18*

4. Vacuum Erection Device **19**

The Device *19*
Technique *20*
Indications *20*
Side Effects *21*
Results *22*

5. Surgery for Erectile Dysfunction **23**

Surgery *23*
Types of Penile Prosthesis *23*
Penile Implant Procedure *24*
Complications of Penile Implant *25*
Perforation and Erosion *27*
Poor Glans Support *27*
Mechanical Complications *28*

6. Peyronie's Disease **29**
Presentation *29*
Pathophysiology *29*
Diagnosis *30*
Medications *30*
Multiple Tunica Albuginea Plication Procedure *32*

7. Priapism **33**
History *33*
Clinical Examination *33*
Investigations *33*
Management *34*
Stuttering Priapism *35*

8. Penile Fracture **36**
Presentation *36*
Causes *37*
Diagnosis *37*
Treatment and Prognosis *37*

9. Premature Ejaculation **38**
Complex Problem *38*
How to Define Premature Ejaculation? *38*
Causative Factors *38*
Management *39*
Certain Other Methods *40*

10. Male Infertility **41**
Hormonal Evaluation (FSH and Testosterone) *41*
Semen Culture *42*
Scrotal Ultrasound and Doppler *43*
Genetic Testing *43*
Management Options for Oats (Non-varicocele Related) *44*
Indications and Techniques for Correcting a Varicocele *45*
Microsurgical Varicocelectomy *45*
Laparoscopy for Varicocelectomy *46*
Additional Investigations *47*
Diagnosis and Management *49*
Testicular Sperm Retrieval *52*
Assisted Reproduction *53*

11. Vasectomy **54**
History *54*
Vasectomy in India *54*
Preoperative Counseling *56*
Complications *57*

12. New Innovations in Fields of Male Infertility **59**
Robots to Cure Male Infertility *59*
Robotic Vasectomy Reversal *60*

13. Andropause—Myth or Reality? **61**
Prevalence *61*
Male Menopause is Reality and can Seriously Compromise Quality of Life *62*

14. Pharmacology in Andrology **63**
Medical Management Overview in Andrology *63*
Intracavernosal Injection of Vasoactive Drugs (ICIVAD) *64*
Idiopathic Oligospermia: Management *65*
Specific Medical Therapy in Oligospermia *65*
Testosterone Replacement Therapy for Androgenization *66*
Drugs Therapy in Premature Ejaculation *67*

15. Setting up an Andrology Suite **70**
Male Impotence *70*
Color-Doppler Ultrasound *72*
Nocturnal Penile Tumescence Rigidity Test *73*
Male Infertility Set up *74*
Surgical Microscope *74*
Sperm Retrieval *76*
Anejaculation *77*
Electroejaculator *77*

16. Understanding Sexual Dysfunction: An Overview **78**
Definition *78*
Revised Classification DSM-5 *78*
Revised Diagnostic Criteria Applicable to all Diagnosis *78*
Traditional Female Sexual Response Cycle *79*
Proposed Intimacy-Based Female Sex Response Cycle *80*
Brief Screening for Female Sexual Dysfunction *86*
Algorithm for Establishing a Diagnosis of Female Sexual Dysfunction *86*
General Treatment Guidelines *87*
Referral for Female Sexual Dysfunction *89*
Basic Treatment Strategies for 'FSD' *89*
Female Sexual Dysfunction—Treatment Option on the Horizon *90*
Diagnostic and Statistical Manual of Mental Disorders DSM-5 2013 *91*
Sexual Dysfunction Assessed in a Survey *92*
Specific Techniques *93*

17. Psychosexual Dysfunction: An Overview **96**
Definition *96*
Causes *96*
Risk Factors *97*
Treatment *98*
Prevention *101*

Index *103*

1 Anatomy and Physiology of the Male Reproductive System

MALE REPRODUCTIVE SYSTEM

The human male reproductive system (Fig. 1.1) includes:

1. Hypothalamic-pituitary-testis axis (Hormonal regulation)
2. Testes, epididymis, vas deferens, seminal vesicles, prostate and urethra (production and transport).

Production of spermatozoa requires approximately 3 months from the initial mitotic divisions through the myriad changes readying sperm for ejaculation and fertilization. It acquires the ability to fertilize as well as a capacity for motility in the epididymis.

ANATOMY OF THE SPERM

The human spermatozoon is approximately 60 μm in length. Normal forms have an oval sperm head, 4.5 μm long and 3 μm wide, consisting principally of a nucleus, which contains the highly compacted chromatin material, and the acrosome, a membrane-bound organelle that covers 40–70% of the surface of the sperm

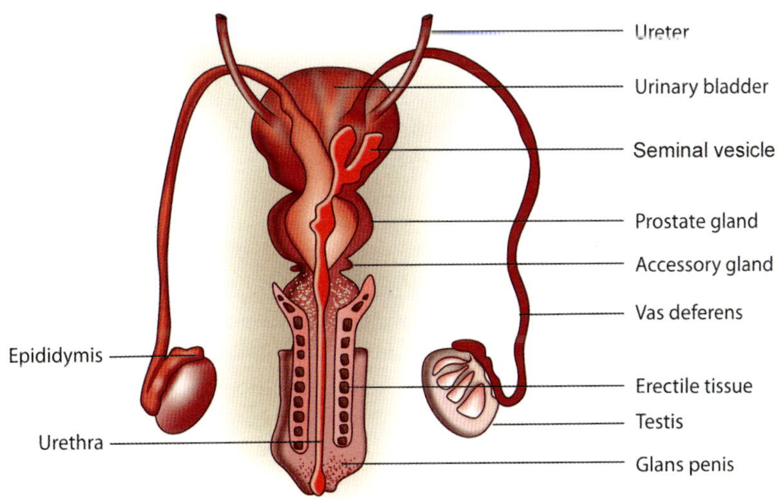

Figure 1.1: Male reproductive system

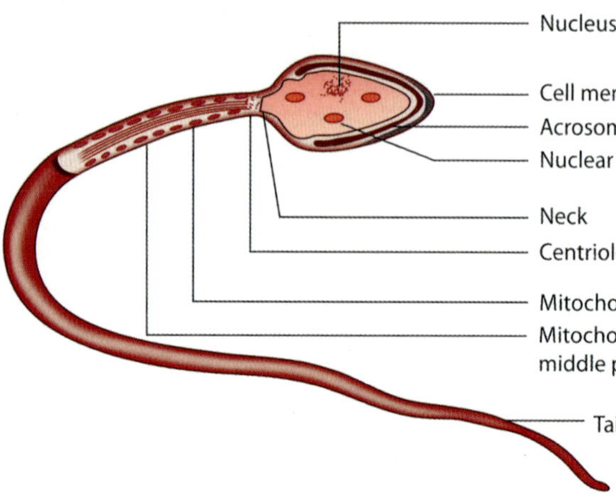

Figure 1.2: Sperm cell

head and contains the enzymes required for penetration of the outer vestments of the egg prior to fertilization. The middle piece of the spermatozoon is a highly organized segment consisting of helically arranged mitochondria surrounding a set of outer dense fibers and the characteristic 9 + 2 microtubular structure of the sperm axoneme. The mitochondria contain the enzymes required for oxidative metabolism and the production of adenosine triphosphate (ATP), the primary energy source for the cell. Absence of some components of the microtubules is associated with immotile cilia in the sinus and pulmonary tracts, with resultant pulmonary and sinus infections. The association of sperm immotility with upper respiratory infections (Young's syndrome) due to ciliary dysfunction or absent dynein cross-arms between the microtubules (Kartagener's syndrome) resulting in bronchiectasis and nonmotile sperm have been well documented (Fig. 1.2).

HORMONAL CONSIDERATIONS

The entire system of hormone balance is initiated by the pulsatile hypothalamic release of gonadotropin-releasing hormone (GnRH). Pituitary luteinizing hormone (LH) secretion is determined by GnRH pulses from the hypothalamus that occur approximately every 2 hours and are carried via a venous portal network to the pituitary. LH and follicle-stimulating hormone (FSH) secretion is stimulated by GnRH. Within the testis, LH stimulates Leydig cell synthesis of testosterone. Testosterone production by the Leydig cell provides locally high intratesticular concentrations of this hormone. It stimulates spermatogenesis. Testosterone concentrations have both age wise and diurnal variations. Testosterone reaches a maximum concentration during the second or third decade of life, then reaches a plateau, and declines thereafter. Testosterone secretion reaches a peak in the morning.

Testosterone is converted intracellularly within most androgen-sensitive organs to dihydrotestosterone; this regulates the prostate, seminal vesicles, vas deferens, and other sex accessory organs.

TESTICULAR ANATOMY

The human testis is an ovoid mass that lies within each hemiscrotum with average volume of 20 cc. Normal longitudinal length of the testis is approximately 3.5–4.5 cm. The testicular parenchyma is surrounded by a capsule containing blood vessels, smooth muscle fibers and nerve fibers sensitive to pressure. The testis contains seminiferous tubules and interstitial cells. The tubules are segregated into regions by connective tissue septa. The seminiferous tubules are long V-shaped tubules, both ends of which usually terminate in the rete testis. Measurement of testicular size is critical in the evaluation of the infertile man, since seminiferous tubules occupy approximately 80% of testicular volume. So, a rough estimate of spermatogenic capacity can be obtained. Testicular consistency is also of value in determining fertility capacity. A soft testis is likely to reflect degenerating spermatogenic components. The seminiferous tubules drain toward the central superior and posterior regions of the testis, the rete testis. The rete coalesces in the superior portion of the testis, just anterior to the testicular vessels, to from 5–10 efferent ductules. These efferent ducts leave the testis and travel to enter caput region of the epididymis. The efferent ducts coalesce to form a single epididymal tubule (Fig. 1.3).

The artery to the testis is specialized in that it is highly coiled and intimately associated with a network of anastomotic veins that form the pampiniform plexus. The counter flowing vessels are separated only by the thickness of their vascular wall in some areas. This vascular arrangement facilitates the exchange of heat. The counter-current exchange of heat in the spermatic cord provides blood to the testis that is 2 to 4°C lower than rectal temperature in the normal individual. A loss of the temperature differential is associated with testicular dysfunction in varicocele or cryptorchidism. **In the distal inguinal canal, 50% of men will have a single testicular artery, with 30% of men having two arteries and 20% with three arteries.**

The spermatic veins are thin-walled; less muscularized, and lack effective valves except at the inflow points into the inferior vena cava or the renal vein.

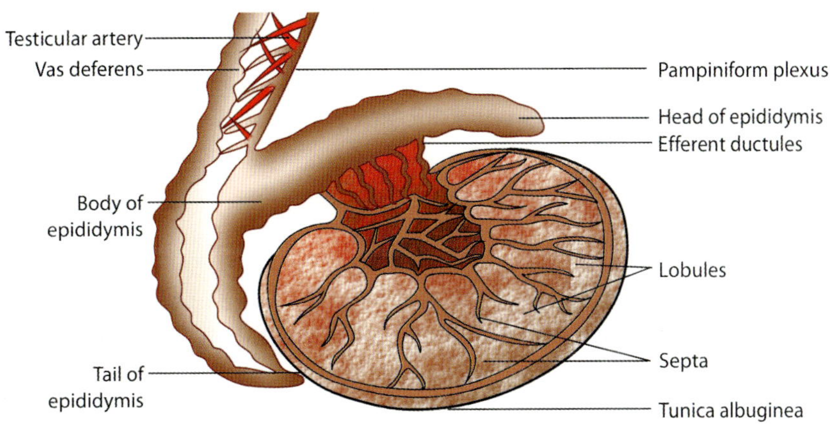

Figure 1.3: Testis, epididymis and vas deferens

The right spermatic vein usually drains into the vena cava. The left spermatic vein drains into the left renal vein. The renal vein on the left side is thought to have a higher intraluminal pressure because the vein is compressed as it passes between the superior mesenteric artery and the aorta (nutcracker effect). This explains to certain extent the higher prevalence of varicoceles on the left side.

SEMINIFEROUS TUBULES

The structures involved in this process include germinal elements and supporting cells—Sertoli cells. The germinal elements comprise a slowly dividing primitive stem cell population, the rapidly proliferating spermatogonia, spermatocytes undergoing meiosis, and the metamorphosing spermatids.

From birth to approximately 7 years of life, there appears to be very little morphological change within the human testis. From 7 to 9 years of life, mitotic activity of gonocytes is detectable, with spermatogonia populating the base of the seminiferous tubule in numbers equal to those of the Sertoli cells. There appears to be little further morphological change in spermatogonia until spermatogenesis begins at the time of puberty.

EPIDIDYMIS

Spermatozoa become functional gametes only after they migrate through the epididymis and undergo an additional maturation process, thereby acquiring the capacities for both progressive motility and fertility. Anatomically, the epididymis can be divided into three regions: the caput, the corpus, and the cauda epididymis.

Ejaculation

The rate of transport of fluid through the vas deferens is not known in the human. Just prior to ejaculation, the testes are brought up close to the abdomen and fluid is rapidly transported through the vas deferens toward the region of the ejaculatory ducts and subsequently into the prostatic urethra. After ejaculation, intravasal fluid is transported back toward the epididymis.

The ejaculatory ducts enter the prostatic urethra just lateral to the verumontanum. In the case of obstruction of the ejaculatory ducts, resection of the floor of the prostate should be performed just lateral to the midline and superior to the verumontanum.

MALE ERECTILE APPARATUS

Penis

The **penis** is a pendulous organ suspended from the front and sides of the pubic arch and containing the greater part of the urethra. In the flaccid condition it is cylindrical in shape, but when erect assumes the form of a triangular prism. It is composed of three cylindrical masses of cavernous tissue bound together by fibrous tissue and covered with skin. Two of the masses are lateral, and are

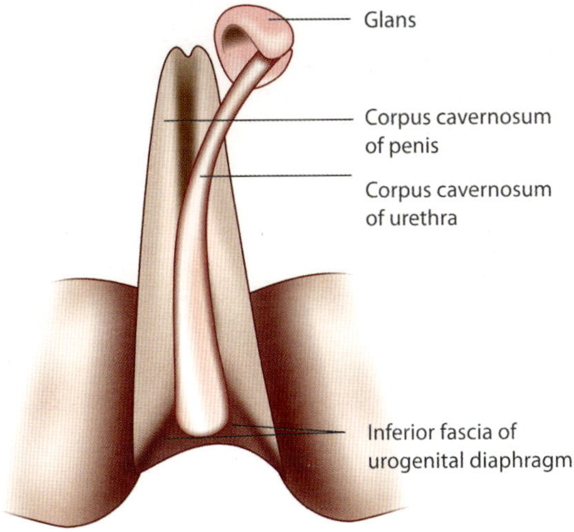

Figure 1.4: The penis

known as the **corpora cavernosa penis;** the third is median, and is termed the **corpus cavernosum urethrae** (Fig. 1.4).

The **corpora cavernosa penis** forms the greater part of the substance of the penis. For their anterior three-fourths they lie in intimate apposition with one another, but behind they diverge in the form of two tapering processes, known as the **crura,** which are firmly connected to the rami of the pubic arch.

The corpora cavernosa penis is surrounded by a strong fibrous envelope consisting of superficial and deep fibers (Tunica albuginea). The superficial fibers are longitudinal in direction, and the deep fibers are arranged circularly around each corpus, and form by their junction in the median plane the **septum of the penis.**

The **corpus cavernosum urethrae** (*corpus spongiosum*) contains the urethra. Behind, it is expanded to form the urethral bulb, and lies in apposition with the inferior fascia of the urogenital diaphragm.

Transverse Section of the Penis

Its anterior end is expanded in the form of the **glans penis,** is moulded on the rounded ends of the corpora cavernosa penis. At the summit of the glans is the slit-like vertical external urethral orifice. The circumference of the base of the glans forms a rounded projecting border, the **corona glandis.**

The **root** (*radix penis*) of the penis is triradiate in form, consisting of the diverging crura, one on either side, or the median urethral bulb. Each crus is covered by the ischiocavernosus, while the bulb is surrounded by the bulbocavernosus. The root of the penis lies in the perineum between the inferior fascia of the urogenital diaphragm and the fascia of Colles'. It is attached to the front of the symphysis pubis by the fundiform and suspensory ligaments which further has attachment to rectus abdominis sheath.

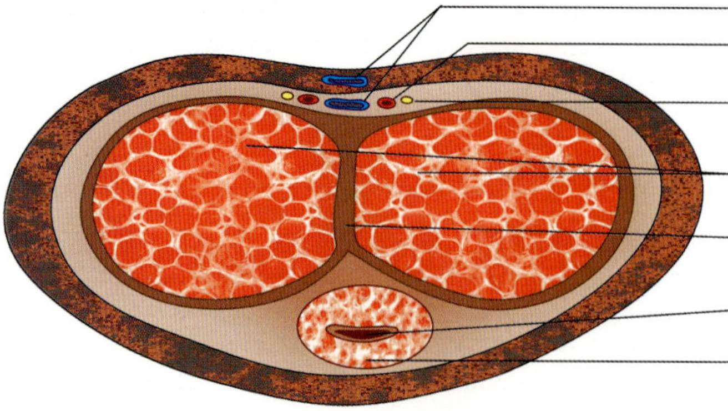

Figure 1.5: Transverse section of penis

Structure of the Penis

From the internal surface of the fibrous envelope of the corpora cavernosa penis, as well as from the sides of the septum, numerous bands or cords are given off, which cross the interior of these corpora cavernosa in all directions, subdividing them into a number of separate compartments, and giving the entire structure a spongy appearance. These bands and cords are called **trabeculae,** and consist of white fibrous tissue, elastic fibers, and plain muscular fibers. In them are contained numerous arteries and nerves (Fig. 1.5).

The fibrous envelope of the corpus cavernosum urethra is thinner, whiter in color, and more elastic than that of the corpora cavernosa penis. The trabeculae are more delicate, nearly uniform in size, and the meshes between them smaller than in the corpora cavernosa penis.

Vessels and nerves: The **arteries** bringing the blood to the cavernous spaces are the deep arteries of the penis and branches from the dorsal arteries of the penis, which perforate the fibrous capsule, along the upper surface, especially near the forepart of the organ. On entering the cavernous structure the arteries divide into branches, which are supported and enclosed by the trabeculae. Some of these arteries end in a capillary network, the branches of which open directly into the cavernous spaces; others assume a tendril-like appearance, and form convoluted and somewhat dilated vessels, which were named by Müller **helicine arteries.**

Arterial Supply of the Penis

The blood from the cavernous spaces is returned by a series of vessels, some of which emerge in considerable numbers from the base of the glans penis and converge on the dorsum of the organ to form the deep dorsal vein; others pass out on the upper surface of the corpora cavernosa and join the same vein; some emerge from the under surface of the corpora cavernosa penis and receiving branches from the corpus cavernosum urethrae, wind around the sides of the penis to end in the deep dorsal vein; but the greater number pass out at the root of the penis and join the prostatic plexus.

The **nerves** are derived from the pudendal nerve and the pelvic plexuses. On the glans and bulb some filaments of the cutaneous nerves have Pacinian bodies connected with them, and, according to Krause, many of them end in peculiar endbulbs.

Erection

Sexual stimulation triggers release of neurotransmitters from the cavernous nerve terminals. This results in relaxation of these smooth muscles and the following events: (1) dilation of the arterioles and arteries by increased blood flow in both the diastolic and systolic phases; (2) trapping of the incoming blood by the expanding sinusoids; (3) compression of the subtunical venous plexuses between the tunica albuginea and the peripheral sinusoids, reducing venous outflow; (4) stretching of the tunica to its capacity, which occludes the emissary veins between the inner circular and outer longitudinal layers and further decreases venous outflow to a minimum; (5) an increase in PO_2 (to about 90 mm Hg) and intracavernous pressure (around 100 mm Hg), which raises the penis from the dependent position to the erect state (the full-erection phase); (6) a further pressure increase (to several hundred millimeters of mercury) with contraction of the ischiocavernosus muscles (rigid-erection phase).

Erectile Dysfunction

2

"Man survives earthquakes, experiences the horrors of illness and all of the tortures of the soul. But the most tormenting tragedy of all time is and will be, the tragedy of the bedroom."

—Tolstoy

Erectile dysfunction (ED) is the inability to achieve and maintain an erection adequate for intercourse to the mutual satisfaction of the man and his partner.

PREVALENCE

The Massachusetts male aging study—52% of men between the ages of 40 and 70 (1987–1997). Erectile dysfunction is classified as minimal, moderate, or complete. Of the 52% of men who suffer from erectile dysfunction, 17% have minimal ED, 25% have moderate ED, and 10% have complete ED.

The worldwide incidence of erectile dysfunction estimated at over 152 million men, with a forecast of 322 million men by the year 2025. This may be because of change in lifestyle-increasing population suffering from metabolic syndrome (syndrome with increased cholesterol, hypertension, cardiac disease, hyperuricemia and diabetes), smoking and substance abuse. It may also be because of increasing stress and change in interpersonal relationships.

PATHOPHYSIOLOGY

- The cGMP: Smooth muscle relaxation and blood flows into the cavernous sinuses and the penis becomes erect.
- At the same time, the veins in the penis are squeezed almost completely shut due to this pressure. Since the veins are shut, blood cannot drain from the penis, and it remains erect.
- Once the arousal has subsided, the cGMP is broken down and the penis again becomes flaccid.
- The main chemical responsible: Phosphodiesterase-5 (PDE-5).
- Sildenafil, Tadalafil are PDE-5 inhibitors: Preventing the breakdown of cGMP, thus keeping blood in the penis to maintain the erection.

CAUSES

Since an erection requires a precise sequence of events, ED can occur when any of the events is disrupted. The sequence includes nerve impulses in the brain, spinal column, and area around the penis, and response in muscles, fibrous tissues, veins, and arteries in and near the corpora cavernosa.

Damage to nerves, arteries, smooth muscles, and fibrous tissues, often as a result of disease, is the most common cause of ED. Erectile dysfunction is usually caused by one or more of the following pathologies:

- *Arterial vascular pathology:* Heart disease and vascular problems also raise the risk of erectile dysfunction.
- *Neurologic pathology*
- *Endocrine causes:* Between 35 and 50% of men with diabetes experience ED. Also aging males can have dropping levels of testosterone which may lead to decreased libido, erectile dysfunction (androgen deficiency of aging male). Men with increased levels of prolactin will also experience erectile dysfunction because of decreased libido.
- *Psychogenic causes:* Experts believe that psychological factors such as stress, anxiety (Performance anxiety), guilt (Previous sexual experiences), depression, low self-esteem, and fear of sexual failure cause 10 to 20% of ED cases.
- *Post-surgical:* (Especially radical prostate and bladder surgery for cancer) can injure nerves and arteries near the penis, causing ED.
- *Local pathology:* Penile curvatures—Peyronie's disease, corporal fibrosis-post-trauma, and surgery, post-priapism may also lead to impotence.
- *Medications/substance abuse:* Many common medicines/drugs/substances-blood pressure drugs, antihistamines, antidepressants, tranquilizers, appetite suppressants, alcohol, tobacco and cimetidine (used for acid peptic disease) can produce ED.

EVALUATION

- Somewhat subjective
- Doctor diagnosis
- Validated questionnaires like IIEF (International Index of Erectile Function).

DIAGNOSIS

Patient History

Medical and sexual histories help define the degree and nature of ED. A medical history can disclose diseases that lead to ED, while a simple recounting of sexual activity might distinguish among problems with sexual desire, painful sex, either difficulty in initiation or maintenance of erection, ejaculatory problems like-retrograde ejaculation or anejaculation, or problems with orgasm—anorgasmia.

Physical Examination

1. A physical examination can give clues to systemic problems. For example, if the penis is not sensitive to touching focal neurological problems can pinpoint to neurological disorders.

2. Abnormal secondary sex characteristics (defective androgenization), such as hair pattern or breast enlargement, can point to hormonal problems, which would mean that the endocrine system is involved.
3. The patient may have circulatory disturbances in the form of decreased pulsations in the ankle/popliteal region.
4. Local pathologies: Penile curvatures, tender penile plaques will reveal local pathological cause for erectile dysfunction.

PRACTICAL TIPS

Psychogenic Causes

1. Younger patient (<40)
2. Preservation of morning erections and nocturnal erections
3. Achieve erection with masturbation
4. May be partner-specific (May achieve erection with specific person-Quoad)
5. Often sudden onset (Related to sudden outburst of stress in life).

Organic Erectile Dysfunction

1. Gradual deterioration over the period of months or years
2. Decrease in morning erections and nocturnal erections
3. No erections with masturbation
4. No loss of libido
5. Presence of comorbid conditions like long standing hypertension, hyperlipidemia or diabetes.

LABORATORY TESTS

Several laboratory tests can help diagnose ED. Tests for systemic diseases include blood counts, urinalysis, lipid profile, and measurements of creatinine and liver enzymes. Measuring the amount of free and total testosterone, thyroid function or prolactin in the blood can yield information about problems with the endocrine system and is indicated especially in patients with decreased sexual desire.

Serum PSA is usually indicated in men over 50 years as if these men require testosterone replacement or supplementation they would need careful follow-up with digital rectal examination and serum PSA to rule out co-existing prostatic carcinoma which may flare up with the administration of testosterone.

OTHER TESTS

Nocturnal Penile Tumescence Tests

Monitoring erections that occur during sleep (nocturnal penile tumescence) can help rule out certain psychological causes of ED. Healthy men have involuntary erections during sleep. If nocturnal erections do not occur, then ED is likely to have a physical rather than psychological cause.

In 1985, the RigiScan was introduced; it was the first device to provide automated, portable NPTR recording. The device combines the monitoring of radial rigidity, tumescence, number, and duration of erectile events with the convenience of a portable system that can be used at home. It consists of a recording unit that can collect data for three separate nights for a maximum of 10 hours each night. The mechanics consist of two loops: one is placed at the base of the penis and the other at the coronal sulcus. By constricting the loops, the device records penile tumescence (circumference) and radial rigidity at the penile base and tip. Measurement (initialization) is first done in the office for 15 to 20 minutes with the patient awake to establish an individual baseline. At home, penile rigidity is registered every 3 minutes by constriction of the loops, applying radial compression. Radial rigidity above 70% represents a non-buckling erection, and a rigidity of less than 40% represents a flaccid penis. The number of erections considered normal is three to six per 8-hour session, lasting an average of 10 to 15 minutes each.

The usual normal NPTR criteria considered are: four to five erectile episodes per night; mean duration longer than 30 minutes; an increase in circumference of more than 3 cm at the base and more than 2 cm at the tip; and maximal rigidity above 70% at both base and tip.

The main advantages of NPT testing are its relative freedom from psychological influences and its ability to detect sleep-related abnormalities. The documented presence of a full erection indicates that the neurovascular axis is functionally intact and that the cause of the ED is most likely psychogenic. Heaton and Morales (1997) have suggested indications for NPTR as follows: (1) suspected sleep disorder; (2) obscure cause of ED; (3) no response to therapy; (4) planned surgical treatment; (5) legally sensitive case; (6) measurement of drug effects in placebo-controlled drug trials; and (7) suspected psychogenic cause.

Color-Doppler Examination

When vascular evaluation is indicated, intracavernous injection with color duplex Doppler ultrasound is the most informative diagnostic test. This may be all that is needed to define and determine severity. Color duplex ultrasound should be used before other tests are considered because it is the least invasive technology for evaluating vascular ED, distinguishing high-from low-flow priapism, and assessing Peyronie's plaque. Recently, the combination of oral sildenafil citrate with visual erotic stimulation has been shown to be an effective noninvasive pharmacologic induction method for penile blood flow evaluation rather than giving intracavernosal injection (which many patients find repulsive at first instance) PSV less than 25 cm/s after intracavernous injection and sexual stimulation has a 100% sensitivity and 95% specificity in selecting patients with abnormal penile arteriography, because it reflects severe cavernous arterial insufficiency. A PSV consistently greater than 35 cm/s is associated with normal arteriography and defines normal cavernous arterial inflow.

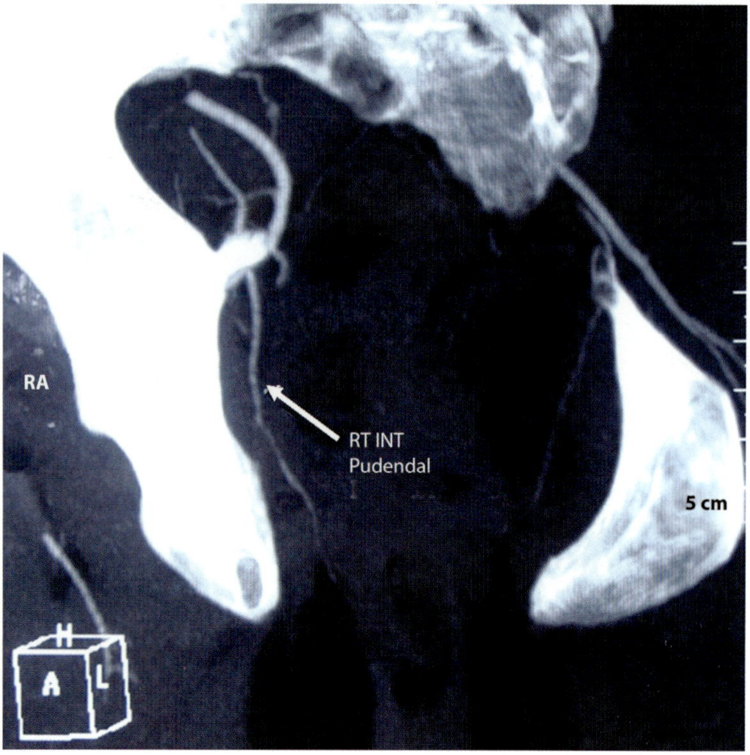

Figure 2.1: Selective internal pudendal angiogram showing pudendal artery stenosis

Penile Arteriography

Arteriography is most useful in providing anatomic information. The inferior epigastric vessels also need to be studied because they are most commonly used for penile revascularization. Because of the high cost and invasive nature of the study, only a small percentage of patients with complex ED are appropriate candidates—ED secondary to a traumatic arterial disruption or in a patient with a history of perineal compression injury. In these highly selected cases, a detailed "road map" of the arterial anatomy is essential to planning surgical reconstruction. Internal Pudental Angiography as shown in Figure 2.1.

Dynamic Infusion Cavernosography and Cavernosometry

This is a complex test done in special circumstances like young men who might be candidates for penile vascular operations, specifically those with a history of pelvic trauma.

Psychosocial Examination

A psychosocial examination, using an interview and a questionnaire, reveals psychological factors. A man's sexual partner may also be interviewed to determine expectations and perceptions during sexual intercourse.

TREATMENT

General Conservative Measures

Most physicians suggest that treatments proceed from least to most invasive. For some men, making a few healthy lifestyle changes may solve the problem. Quitting smoking, losing excess weight, and increasing physical activity may help some men regain sexual function. Avoiding drugs with harmful side effects is considered next. For example, drugs for high blood pressure like thiazides can be changed and alternative medications can be given.

Psychotherapy

Experts often treat psychologically based ED using techniques that decrease the anxiety associated with intercourse. The patient's partner can help with the techniques, which include gradual development of intimacy and stimulation. Master and Johnson's therapy involving couples can solve problems with performance anxiety/premature ejaculation.

Drug Therapy

Drugs for treating ED can be taken orally, injected directly into the penis, or inserted into the urethra at the tip of the penis. In March 1998, the Food and Drug Administration (FDA) approved Viagra, the first pill to treat ED. Since that time, vardenafil hydrochloride (Levitra) and tadalafil (Cialis) have also been approved. Additional oral medicines are being tested for safety and effectiveness. Viagra, Levitra, and Cialis all belong to a class of drugs called phosphodiesterase (PDE) inhibitors. Taken an hour before sexual activity, these drugs work by enhancing the effects of nitric oxide, a chemical that relaxes smooth muscles in the penis during sexual stimulation and allows increased blood flow (Fig. 2.2).

While oral medicines improve the response to sexual stimulation, they do not trigger an automatic erection as injections do. The recommended dose for Sildenafil is 50 mg, and the physician may adjust this dose to 100 mg or 25 mg, depending on the patient. The recommended dose for either Tadalafil is 10 mg, and the physician may adjust this dose to 20 mg if 10 mg is insufficient. A lower dose of 5 mg is available for patients who take other medicines or have conditions that may decrease the body's ability to use the drug.

None of these PDE inhibitors should be used more than once a day. Men who take nitrate-based drugs such as nitroglycerin for heart problems should not use either drug because the combination can cause a sudden drop in blood pressure. Also patients have severe cardiac diseases like recent myocardial infarction; reduced stress tolerance should avoid PDE-5 inhibitors.

Many men achieve stronger erections by injecting drugs into the penis, causing it to become engorged with blood (Fig. 2.3). Drugs such as papaverine hydrochloride, phentolamine, and alprostadil (marketed as Caverject) widen blood vessels. These drugs may create unwanted side effects, however, including

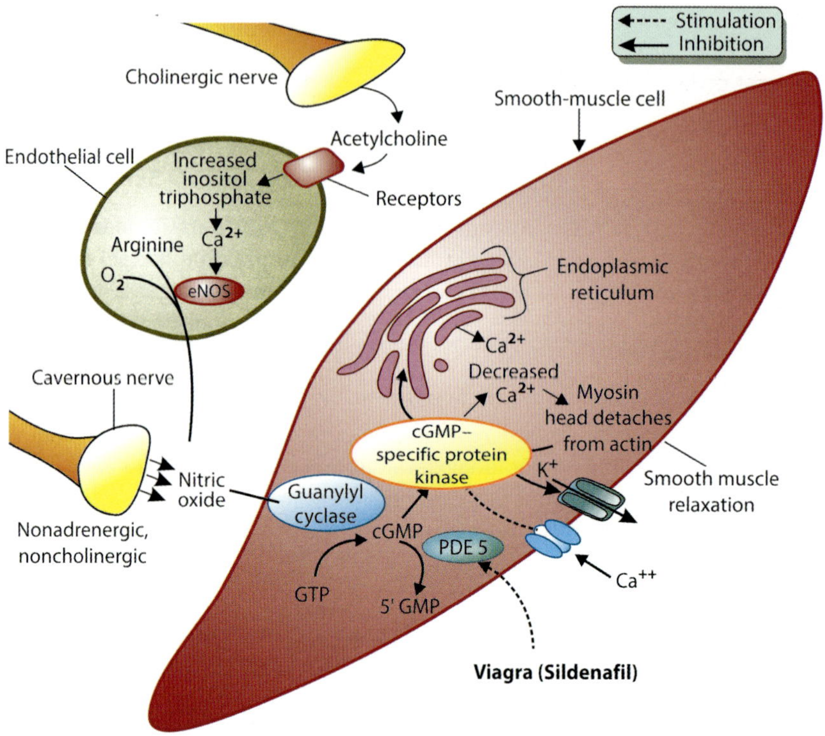

Figure 2.2: Mechanism of action of Viagra like drugs (PDE-5 inhibitors)

pain (36%) persistent erection (4%) and scarring. It gives a success rate of 70–90% but these injections have a drop-out rate of 25–60% because of mainly pain or sometimes development of corporal fibrosis. A system for inserting a pellet of alprostadil into the urethra is marketed as muse. The system uses a prefilled applicator to deliver the pellet about an inch deep into the urethra. An erection will begin within 8–10 minutes and may last 30–60 minutes. The most common side effects are aching in the penis, testicles, and area between the penis and rectum; warmth or burning sensation in the urethra; redness from increased blood flow to the penis; and minor urethral bleeding or spotting.

Vacuum Devices

Mechanical vacuum devices cause erection by creating a partial vacuum, which draws blood into the penis, engorging and expanding it. The devices have three components: a plastic cylinder, into which the penis is placed; a pump, which draws air out of the cylinder; and an elastic band, which is placed around the base of the penis to maintain the erection after the cylinder is removed and during intercourse by preventing blood from flowing back into the body. The

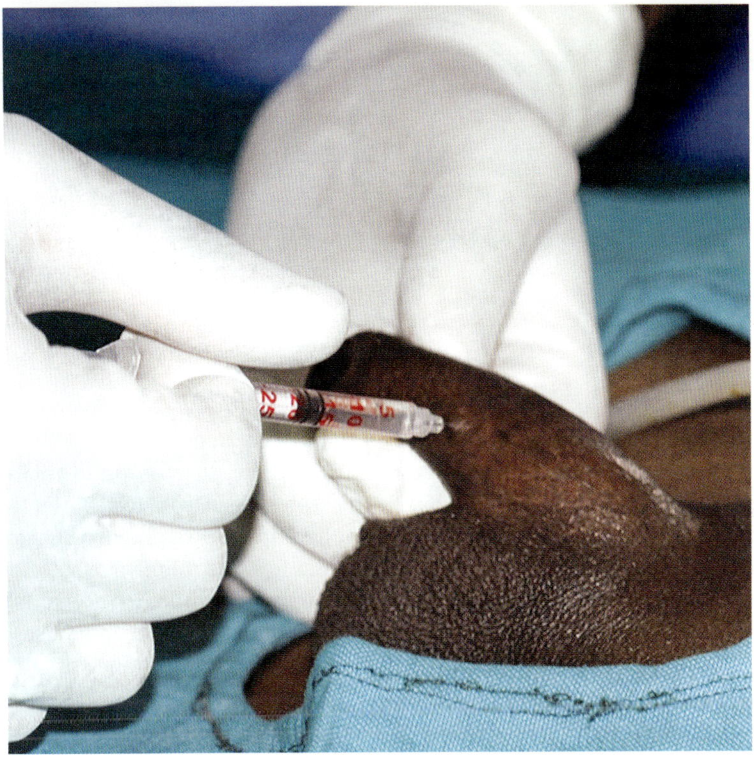

Figure 2.3: Intracorporal injection of vasoactive substances: Note the site of injection

satisfaction rate varies from 35–80% but the problems with the vacuum erection devices are—cold penis, loosely hanging penis, sometimes it can lead to bruises especially patient using it roughly and on aspirin or clopidogrel.

Intracavernosal Injection

3

INTRACAVERNOSAL INJECTION OF VASOACTIVE DRUGS—PRACTICAL APPROACH

One of the most dramatic changes in urology has been the introduction of intracavernous injection of vasoactive drugs for the diagnosis and treatment of ED. At the 1983 annual meeting of the American Urological Association, Brindley personally demonstrated erection after injection of phenoxybenzamine (with much surprise and shock to the audience). Subsequently, Zorgniotti and Lefleur (1985) reported their experience instructing patients in the technique of autoinjection of a mixture of papaverine and phentolamine for home use.

Intracavernosal injections provide an effective therapy for men with erectile dysfunction who cannot take oral agents or for whom oral agents are not effective.

DRUGS AND PATHOPHYSIOLOGY

Papaverine

Papaverine, an alkaloid isolated from the opium poppy, exerts an inhibitory effect on PDE, leading to increased cyclic AMP and cyclic GMP in penile erectile tissue. Papaverine also blocks voltage-dependent calcium channels, thus impairing calcium influx and it may also impair calcium-activated potassium and chloride currents. All these actions relax cavernous smooth muscle and penile vessels. Papaverine is metabolized in the liver and the plasma half-life is 1 to 2 hours.

Alprostadil (Prostaglandin E_1)

Alprostadil is the synthetic form of a naturally occurring fatty acid (i.e. alprostadil refers to the exogenous form, PGE_1 to the endogenous compound). It causes smooth muscle relaxation, vasodilation and inhibition of platelet aggregation through elevation of intracellular cyclic AMP. Alprostadil is metabolized by the enzyme prostaglandin-15-hydroxydehydrogenase, which has been shown to be active in human corpus cavernosum. After intracavernous injection, 96% of alprostadil is locally metabolized within 60 minutes and no change in peripheral blood levels has been observed.

How to Give Injection

The injection may be given anywhere from the base of the penis to two-thirds of the way down the penile shaft at the 10 o'clock and 2 o'clock locations on the upper side of the penis away from the urethra and the head of the penis. Injections are rotated within that area and the side of the injection is alternated with each injection.

PATHOPHYSIOLOGY

Preparation

Methodology: Start with 29–30 G Insulin syringe for the injection therapy.

Papaverine: It can be started with 15 and given till 60 mg. Inject in any corpus.

Bimix: Add chlorpromazine (4 ml papavarine to 0.1 ml chlorpromazine combination) start with 0.1 to 0.2 ml and then gradually increased. Again the injection can be given in any one of the corpus.

Kulkarni VR, Shah RS, Gupte DM, Mehte MK. A clinical study of the erection-inducing effects of intracavernosal chlorpromazine. *Int J Imp Res 1996.*

Trimix: Add PGE-150 mcg (conventional vial contains 500 mcg so we will have to take 0.1 ml).

Procedure

1. Start in lying down position.
2. Give complete privacy.
3. Ask patient to fantasize and stroke his penis (patient allowed to read erotic materials).
4. If no response after 15 minutes ask him to stand erect and repeat the procedure.
5. Some men are known to have late response so minimum wait till 30–45 minutes advisable.
6. If no benefit call the patient at next sitting and increase the dose.

HOME ADMINISTERED INJECTION

1. If the diagnostic testing helps then patient is started on home administered injection. Refilled insulin syringes can be given. This can be stored at room temperature for 6 months.
2. Good sexual counseling and involvement of female partner is essential.
3. Sometimes obese person cannot do it on his own so wife can give injection while husband stretches the penis.
4. The patient has to be warned about priapism. It is always good for patient to have access to the andrologist for any complications.
5. As priapism is rare the patient needs reassurance and first 2–3 injections can be started in clinic to gain confidence and allay fears about the injection.

PATIENT ACCEPTANCE AND DROP-OUT

In long-term studies, 13–60% of patients drop-out for a number of reasons. These include loss of interest, loss of partner, poor erectile response, penile pain, concomitant illness (Many obese individuals are reluctant for injection because abdominal fat apron prevents them good vision of the penis. And the partner initially may help but later on gives up thinking this as more of mechanical process than romantic emotional encounter), recovery of spontaneous erection and ultimate choice of other therapy (Many people in the interim go for penile implant without having to resort to injection every time they have sexual act).

SERIOUS ADVERSE EFFECTS

Priapism and fibrosis are the two more serious side effects associated with intracavernosal injection therapy. Some people face pain on injection and this can be a reason for abandoning the injection therapy.

Vacuum Erection Device

4

Vacuum erection devices, also known as vacuum constriction devices have been utilized for improving erectile rigidity for over a century. In its current form it has gained popularity only over the past twenty years. It has been FDA approved for use in the management of men with erectile dysfunction (ED). There are a number of medical equipment companies that have specially-designed devices which are carefully constructed so that a limited amount of pressure is allowed to develop. This is to reduce the likelihood of pressure-induced penile injury. This pressure is approximately 200–250 mm Hg.

THE DEVICE

The vacuum device consists of a clear plastic cylinder with an aperture at one end that is placed over the penile shaft. At the other end of the cylinder is a pump mechanism that is used to generate negative pressure within the cylinder. The pump mechanism can be in the form of either a manually operated or a battery-operated system (Fig. 4.1). The former generally requires two hands to control the

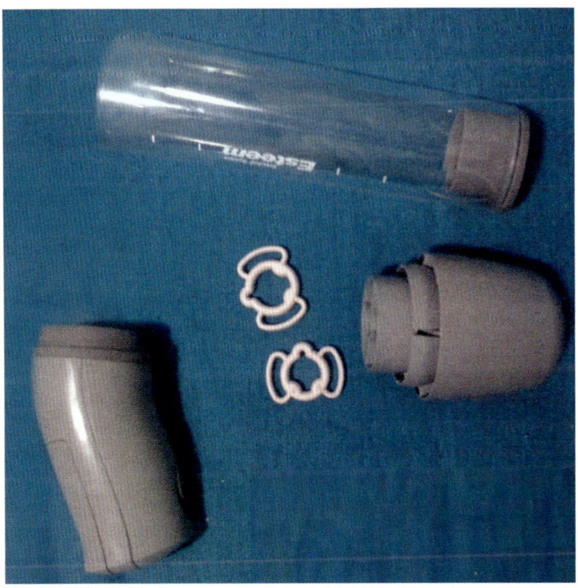

Figure 4.1: Vacuum erection device

device, one on the pump handle and the other to steady the cylinder on the penis itself. The battery-operated device can be used with one hand. In this system, the trigger mechanism is on the top end of the cylinder and thus one hand can activate the pump and steady the cylinder at the same time. This is an important consideration for patients with poor manual dexterity or strength, such as men with Parkinson's disease or rheumatoid arthritis. All FDA approved cylinders have pop-off valves, which limit the amount of pressure held within the chamber.

TECHNIQUE

Once a decision has been made to pursue sexual relations, water-soluble jelly is applied to the base of the penis. This maneuver prevents air from seeping into the chamber, by creating a water-tight seal, thus maintaining the negative pressure within the cylinder. Some men may find that trimming the pubic hair may aid achieving this water-tight seal. Once the cylinder has been placed over the penile shaft and held firmly against the pubic bone, the pump mechanism can be activated (either by hand or battery). Slow generation of the negative pressure prevents penile pain due to too rapid a build-up of pressure within the cylinder. The negative pressure causes an inflow of blood into the corporal bodies, both arterial and venous in nature. The latter blood is drawn into the erectile chambers in a retrograde fashion.

Many men find that double-pumping increases the comfort level. This technique involves the generation of negative pressure and then letting some of the negative pressure off, waiting a while and then recommencing with the negative pressure build-up and repeating the process until a full erection is achieved. Early on in a patients experience with the vacuum device, this technique is to be encouraged until the patient develops a comfort level with the amount of negative pressure that he can tolerate and that gives him a functional erection. Once the erection has been achieved, a constriction ring (band) must be applied to the base of the penis to act as an artificial valve, thus maintaining the blood within the corporal bodies. The rings come in a variety of shapes, sizes, and most importantly tension (tightness). Trial and error is used to define which ring size is most comfortable and efficient. Most manufacturers suggest that the constriction ring remain in place for no longer than 30 minutes. Once the ring is in place the plastic cylinder can be removed and sexual relations may commence.

INDICATIONS

The vacuum device is indicated for men with ED. There are no specific conditions that would interfere with the use of these devices. However, caution should be exercised by men if they are: (i) using blood-thinners or have a history of bleeding disorders, (ii) have diminished penile sensation, (iii) have significant penile curvature, or (iv) have a history of priapism (prolonged erection) or are at risk for its development (see section on *Priapism*). Anticoagulant therapy may cause the patient to develop bruising and swelling in the penis due to rupture of the superficial veins on the shaft of the penis resulting from the constriction ring. In the patient who is not on anticoagulant therapy this trauma is uncommon and if it occurs usually resolves of its own accord. Given this, we avoid the use of a vacuum device in this patient population. Likewise, patients with a history of bleeding disorders should be directed toward other treatments.

Patients who have reduced sensation in their penis, especially men with spinal cord injury, are at risk for trauma with repeated use of the constriction band. It should be used with extreme caution in this group and the ring should be applied for only short periods of time. Men with Peyronie's disease (acquired penile curvature) or congenital penile curvature, with significant degrees of curvature should be discouraged from using a vacuum device as the straight cylinder may exert significant stress on the curved penis resulting in trauma to the already bent shaft of the penis. Patients with hematologic forms of *venocclusive* priapism (sickle cell disease, thalassemia, or leukemia) should not use a vacuum device under any circumstances.

The above patient groups represent just a tiny fraction of all patients who present for the evaluation and treatment of ED. The VED is a simple and safe form of impotence therapy. It typically receives good insurance coverage and most importantly, it is totally reversible. If the patient does not wish to continue with this therapy, it is easily stopped and if used in a proper fashion no long-term negative effects will have occurred. It has minimal disadvantages. It is easy to use, although we suggest to all of our patients to spend one visit in clinic to be formally and properly educated regarding its optimum use. We have found that patients acceptance and compliance increase with this approach. However, there are a significant number of patients who find this treatment option unacceptable. Many feel this way because of two important factors, namely cosmetics and difficulty integrating this technique into love-making. In the white male the inflow of blood combined with the application of a constriction band renders the penis cool in temperature and causes a large amount of superficial vein swelling. These factors make the vacuum device erection a non-cosmetic one and the younger patient and the impotent patient who is currently not in a stable long-term relationship often find this unacceptable. It has been estimated that the surface temperature of the penis during use of the VED is 1C lower than the temperature prior to application of the device. The patient and his partner should be counseled regarding this fact prior to the initial use of the device. The average man using such a device will typically take 10–20 minutes to obtain a significant erection of penetration rigidity. This time combined with the mechanical nature of the treatment modality makes this option cumbersome for some men and they may have some difficulty integrating it into sexual relations.

SIDE EFFECTS

Bruising, skin breakdown and penile pain associated with the application of the constriction band have already been discussed. The tightness of the band may also result in failure to achieve an ejaculation (although no interference with orgasm should occur) and the development of a temporary penile numbness.

One of the other problems with the erection achieved with the vacuum device is that it may hinge at the point of application of the constriction ring. That is, the penis behind the ring is soft and only that portion of the shaft that is beyond the ring has any degree of hardness. Therefore, the ring must be applied as far towards the base of the penis as possible.

RESULTS

Despite the apparent drawbacks to the use of vacuum devices, there is a population of patients who find its use easy and it has allowed many couples to successfully resume penetrative sexual relations. A number of reports have cited satisfaction rates above 80%. This treatment has been shown to result in definite improvement in erection hardness, increase in frequency of sex and increase in overall sexual satisfaction. Increased satisfaction for the partner has also been demonstrated. Drop-out rates of up to 30% have been cited and the most common reasons for drop-out include inadequate rigidity, penile pain, failure to ejaculate and dissatisfaction with penile appearance and temperature. The vacuum device is suitable for all groups of patients with ED except those listed as contraindications above. Patients should be comprehensively counseled regarding the pros and cons of this modality. Furthermore, patients should not be just sent home with a video to watch, they should have in-office counseling by a health care worker experienced in the working of the device. This approach maximizes patient acceptance, satisfaction and long-term compliance. In the era of oral therapy, the vacuum device is currently viewed as a second-line therapy, one which, however, has good patient/partner satisfaction and an excellent safety profile.

Surgery for Erectile Dysfunction

5

SURGERY

Surgery usually has one of three goals:

1. To implant a device that can cause the penis to become erect (penile implant surgery)
2. To reconstruct arteries to increase flow of blood to the penis (penile revascularization surgery for patient with focal arterial stenosis-post-trauma)
3. To block off veins that allow blood to leak from the penile tissues (penile venous leak-particularly detected on Doppler showing persistence end-diastolic velocity more than 5 cm/sec).

Implanted devices, known as prostheses, can restore erection in many men with ED. The patient who do not respond to intracavernosal injection of vasodilator agents or Vacuum Erection Device. Neophallus reconstructed patients are also candidates for penile implant surgery. The contraindications for the penile implant are uncontrolled diabetes, spinal cord injury patients, and patients with severe psychiatric imbalance, neurogenic bladder and very short penis. The implant gives erection with causing some decrease in length so this thing has to be emphasized to the patient before the surgery.

TYPES OF PENILE PROSTHESIS

A. *Non-inflatable (Malleable, hinged prosthesis):* Less costly but gives constant erection and needs special clothing for concealment of the erection.
B. *Inflatable (2 pieces and 3 pieces variety):* Expensive, surgery is technically demanding but gives near to normal erection.

Choice of Three-Piece Implants

American Medical System (AMS)

- 700CX: Diameter 12 to 18 mm length constant.
- 700 ultrex: Girth 12 to 18 mm, length increases. So to a patient concerned about the length of the penis postimplant this is a good choice.
- 700 with inhibizone coating.

Mentor Coloplast

Mentor alpha 1: 12–22 cm length for normal corpora.

Mentor titan narrow: For fibrosed/narrow corporae.

Mentor titan OTR: One touch release valve for easier usage.

Description of Inflatable Implant

Inflatable implants consist of paired cylinders, which are surgically inserted inside the penis and can be expanded using pressurized fluid. Tubes connect the cylinders to a fluid reservoir and a pump, which are also surgically implanted. The patient inflates the cylinders by pressing on the small pump, located under the skin in the scrotum. Inflatable implants can expand the length and width of the penis. They also leave the penis in a more natural state when not inflated.

Advantages with the Penile Implants

- Good rigidity
- Freedom from medications
- Outpatient/24 hr surgery
- Resume sexual activity 4–6 weeks
- No loss of ability to ejaculate or achieve orgasm.

Surgery to repair arteries can reduce ED caused by obstructions that block the flow of blood. The best candidates for such surgery are young men with discrete blockage of an artery because of an injury to perineum or fracture of the pelvis.

Surgery to veins that allow blood to leave the penis usually involves an opposite procedure-intentional blockage. Blocking off veins (ligation) can reduce the leakage of blood that diminishes the rigidity of the penis during erection. However, the results are not long lasting so the venous ligation surgery have diminished.

PENILE IMPLANT PROCEDURE

Equipment needed:

- Scott retractor, hook retractors
- Small deavers
- Hegars dilators
- Furlow inserter with Keith needle
- Metzenbaum scissors

Procedure Steps

- Silicon Foleys 14 Fr inserted
- Penoscrotal incision is made
- Tunica albuginea of the both corpora exposed
- A 4 cm long longitudinal corporotomy done with stab knife and Metzenbaum scissors

- Corporal dilatation done progressively with Hegars dilators
- Direction of dilatation done laterally to avoid cross perforation of the other corpora and the urethral injury
- Both corpora are continuously irrigated with antibiotic solution
- The distal dilatation is done till the tip of the dilator is felt through the glans to avoid underdilatation and SST deformity
- With the help of ureteric catheter, the corporal length is measured and a suitable implant is chosen
- Sterile saline is cycled through connected corporal cylinders and the pump taking care to avoid any air bubbles (Fig. 5.1A)
- With Furlow inserter, Keith needle is pushed through the glans and along with it the cylinder of the implant is pulled so as to place it in corpora (Fig. 5.1B)
- Both cylinders are placed in the corpora and the pump is placed in the subdartos pouch
- We place the prefilled reservoir in retropubic space through a separate lower abdominal incision
- All the connections are made; a trial inflation and deflation of the implant is carried out
- The two corporotomies are closed with 2-0 Vicryl sutures and the procedure is completed by closing the skin. We do not keep any drain and give a light compressive dressing.
- We keep the catheter for 24 hours
- The penile implant is activated after a period of 6 weeks. The initial few sessions are spent teaching the patient how to inflate and deflate the implant. As corpora gets dilated; the pain during inflation gradually comes down.

COMPLICATIONS OF PENILE IMPLANT

Infection (5–14%)

Infections occurring after penile prosthesis implantation are either early (in the first few weeks following implantation) or late (6 months to 1 or 2 years after implantation). The former are often associated with gram-negative bacteria (70%), whereas the later are usually associated with gram-positive bacteria such as *Staphylococcus epidermidis (30%).* Early infections are usually acquired during the surgery. 56% of cases occur within 6 months, 36% occur within 7–12 months and 2.3% after 5 months.

Preoperatively cephalosporins and aminoglycosides should be administered and postoperatively quinolones should be given.

Early infections are likely to be evident by swelling, erythema, tenderness, possible purulent drainage, and occasionally fever. Late infections may be manifested only by persistent or recurrent long-term pain.

Treatment of a prosthetic infection with appropriate antibiotics usually results in clinical improvement; however, antibiotic treatment rarely permanently eradicates this type of infection. This is thought to be due to harboring of micro-organisms within a biofilm that is adherent to the device. For this reason, when

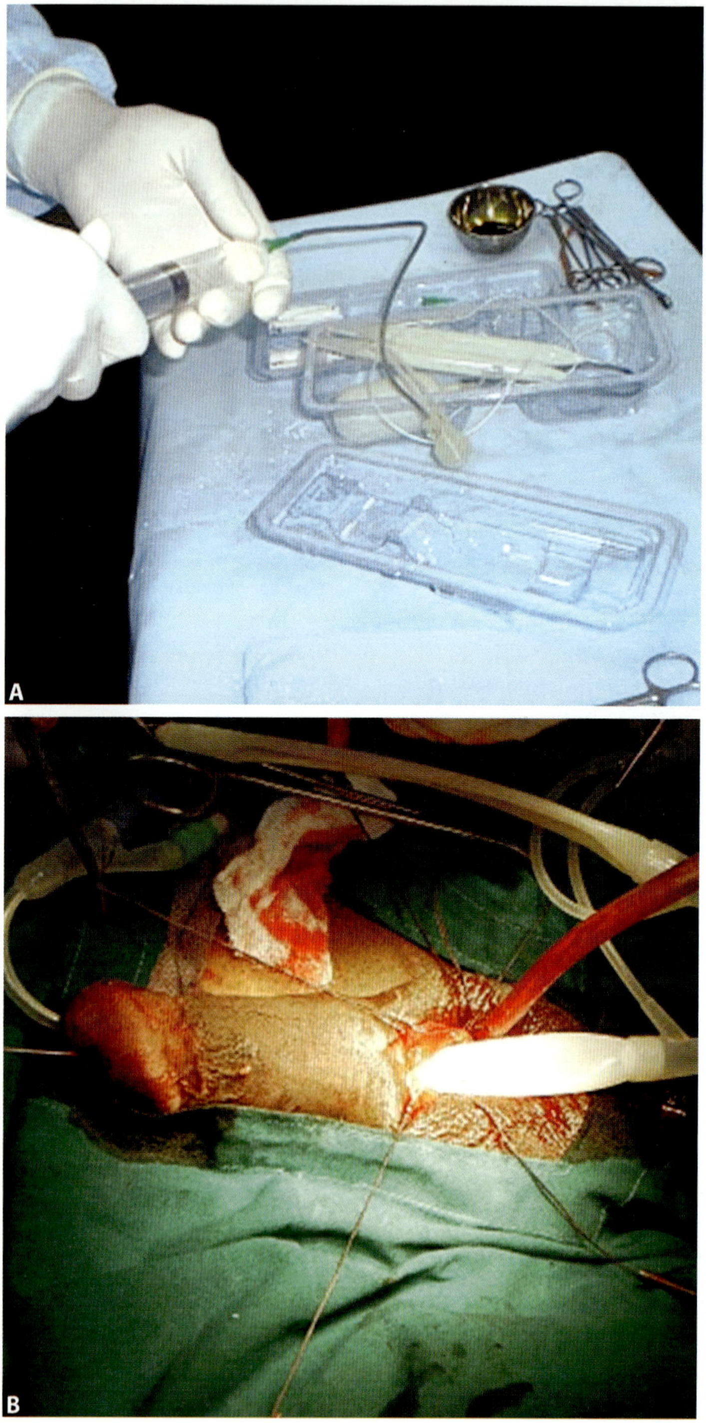

Figures 5.1A and B: Photographs of penile implant surgery being done

a prosthetic infection is present, all components of the prosthesis should be removed. In case of overt infection; the corporal spaces should be lavaged with antibiotic solutions. Vancomycin and Gentamicin are preferentially be used for lavage. After the infection has come into control usually in the interim period the Vacuum Erection Device should be encouraged. The advantage being the VED will cause stretching the corpora and to certain extent increase the length and the girth of the penis and cause easier dilatation during the second surgery. When all incisions have healed and postoperative edema has resolved (usually 2 to 3 months after device removal), reimplantation is advised because early fibrosis is easier to dilate and the scar contraction that leads to shortening has not yet occurred. New Inhibizone implants have come with antibiotics—Rifampicin and Minocycline.

PERFORATION AND EROSION

Perforation is an event that occurs intraoperatively; whereas erosion is an event that occurs or is recognized only postoperatively. When the surgeon is dilating the proximal corpora (crura), a sudden give of the dilator suggests that the crus has been perforated on its medial aspect near its attachment to the pelvic bone. The dilator, usually a smaller size, travels out into the soft tissues of the perineum. Wind Sock correction with Gore-Tex patch is a remedy but rarely necessary. The small area of perforation usually heals over if the proximal part of the implant stays inside the crus.

With distal dilation, crossover to the opposite side may occur or the urethra may be perforated. If urethral perforation occurs, the implant procedure should be abandoned and a urethral catheter should be left in for 7 to 10 days. Prosthesis reimplantation may be done at a later date. To avoid urethral perforation, the surgeon should keep the tip of the dilator under the dorsolateral surface of the corpus cavernosum.

Erosion of the distal end of the prosthesis may occur into the urethra, in which case it is visible through the meatus. This occurs more commonly after semirigid rod implantation, presumably because of constant internal pressure from the rod device. It also occurs more commonly in men with spinal cord injury/diabetic sensory neuropathy because of their lack of sensation. In the case of urethral erosion, a urethral catheter is placed for 10 days to allow urethral healing. Many patients are able to have adequate coitus with only one rod in place; hence, a procedure to reimplant the second rod is usually not necessary. Distal perforations should lead to abandoning the procedure for reimplantation later.

POOR GLANS SUPPORT

Poor support of the glans penis by cylinder or rod tips leads to a drooping appearance of the glans, which is commonly referred to as the SST deformity after the **S**uper**s**onic **T**ransport (Concorde) nose appearance on take off and landing. This deformity may result from inadequate distal dilation, too short cylinders, or, in the case of minor deformity, variations in anatomy. The dorsal plication of the glans back onto the shaft of the penis can be performed.

MECHANICAL COMPLICATIONS

Autoinflation or mechanical failure is a possibility. The average duration of the implant before mechanical failure may be 5–10 years. Replacement is the only solution. Auto-inflation is annoying problem but Mentor has come-up with a reservoir with a lock-out valve. Initial experience with this device suggests that it reduces the incidence of this complication.

6 Peyronie's Disease

Peyronie's disease is characterized by a plaque, or hard lump, that forms within the penis. The plaque, a flat plate of scar tissue, develops in the tunica albuginea part of the penis, which is a covering of the erectile tissues. This condition was described by Fallopius in 1561 and popularized by Gigot De La Peyronie in 1743.

The average age of onset of the disease is 53 years and its prevalence is 3.2% in sexually active men.

PRESENTATION

Cases of Peyronie's disease range from mild to severe. Symptoms may develop slowly or appear overnight. In severe cases, the hardened plaque reduces flexibility, causing pain and forcing the penis to bend or arc during erection. In many cases, the pain decreases over time, but the chordee may remain a problem, making sexual intercourse difficult. The sexual problems that result can disrupt a couple's physical and emotional relationship and can lower a man's self-esteem. Natural history of the disease goes through an active phase of painful erection and changing plaque configuration followed by a secondary phase of painless deformity and progressive calcification. The disease is progressive in 30–40% cases and stable in 40–50% but the spontaneous resolution is rare.

About 30% of men with Peyronie's disease develop other fibrotic disorders as Dupuytren's contracture of the hand. Familial association, diabetes and urethral instrumentation are other causes for Peyronie´s disease.

PATHOPHYSIOLOGY

The trauma is believed to be central reason behind the Peyronie's disease. The trauma to the penis causes buckling of the area of the attachment of the central septum with the tunica albuginea causing rupture of the blood vessesls. The hematoma is accompanied by the accumulation of the inflammatory mediators. The Peyronie's disease goes through three stages:

Step 1: Inflammatory exudates between cavernosa and albuginea consisting of lymphocytes macrophages, plasma cells which secrete active cytokines TGF β1. The TGF β1 increases collagen synthesis, proteoglycans, fibronectin.

Step 2: Fibrous infiltration of the sub tunical layer.

Step 3: Extensive localized fibrosis and ossification.

The plaque causes chordee and venous leak which causes erectile dysfunction. iNOS deficiency is also supposed to be cause behind erectile dysfunction.

DIAGNOSIS

Doctors can usually diagnose Peyronie's disease based on a physical examination. The plaque can be felt when the penis is limp. The erection may be induced by injecting intracavernosal papaverine or bimix and a Doppler ultrasound scan of the penis to pinpoint the location and calcification of the plaque and concomitant venous leak may be done. A photograph may be taken to document the angle of chordee prior to surgical treatment.

MEDICATIONS

The goal of therapy:

1. To restore and maintain the ability to have intercourse.
2. To decrease the pain.
3. To allay the fears in mind of the patient and re-educate him about the disease.
4. To restore cosmetic appearance.

Experts usually recommend surgery only in long-term cases in which the disease is stabilized and the deformity prevents intercourse.

Medical Treatments

Various medications like vitamin E 400 mg three times a day for 3 months, Colchicine 0.5 mg 2 BD for 3 months or Tamoxifen 20 mg BD for 3 months. The placebo controlled trials have not shown efficacy of the medications but colchicines there are no placebo studies. It seems to be effective.

Researchers have also tried injecting chemical agents such as verapamil, collagenase, steroids, and interferon alpha-2b directly into the plaques. Verapamil and interferon alpha-2b seem to diminish curvature of the penis. The other injectable agent, collagenase, is undergoing clinical trial and results are not yet available. Steroids like triamcinolone have caused loss and atrophy of the local tissues and weakening of the tunica. The surgical planes also become difficult after steroid injection.

The intralesional injections are given with 24 G needle making multiple passes through the plaque. There is a possibility that the multiple passes make the plaque weak by mechanical disruption.

Surgery

Three surgical procedures for Peyronie's disease are done for curvature more than 45 degrees in angle making sexual intercourse difficult. Various procedures have been followed like plication (problem of further shortening penis), incision or excision and grafting (tunica vaginalis or saphenous vein graft) or implantation of penile prosthesis.

If the implant alone does not straighten the penis, implantation is combined with one of the other two surgical procedures.

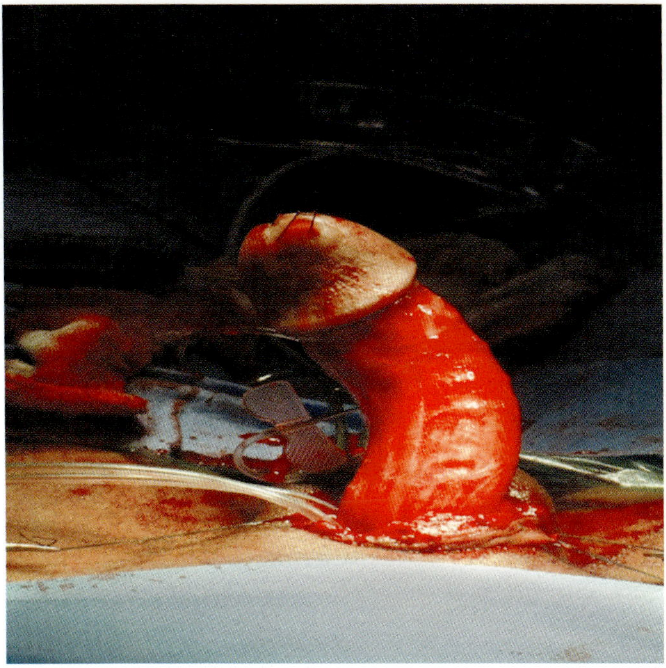

Figure 6.1: Artificial erection and determining the site of maximum curvature

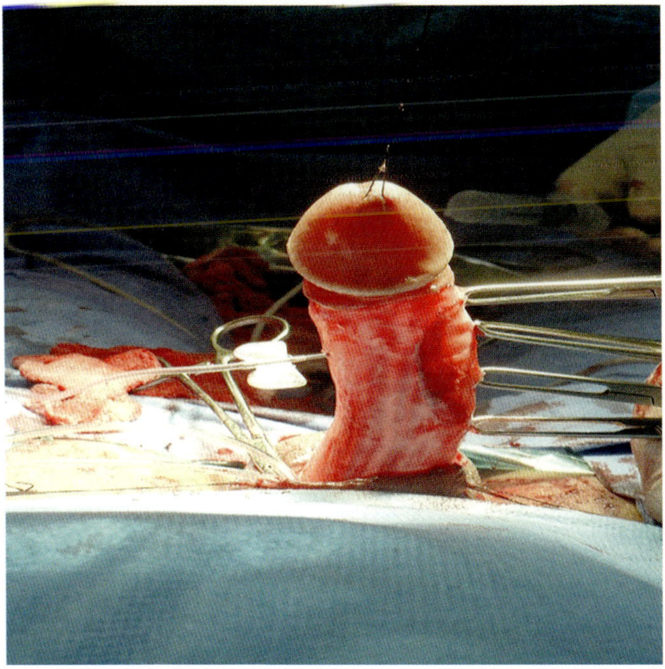

Figure 6.2: Application of Alli's forceps to the tunica albuginea at multiple levels and straightening the curvature

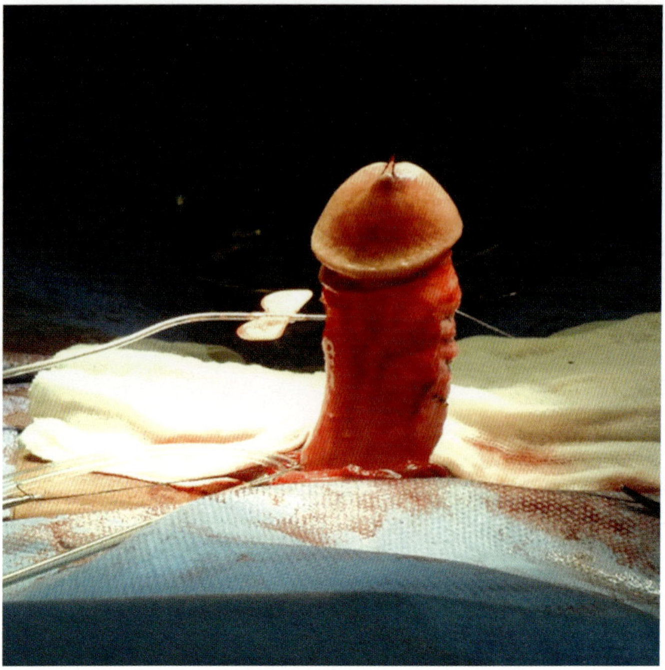

Figure 6.3: Taking the multiple inverted non-absorbable sutures and correcting the chordee

MULTIPLE TUNICA ALBUGINEA PLICATION PROCEDURE

- A circumferential subcoronal incision is made and the penis is degloved till the root. A tourniquet is then placed at the root of the penis.
- An artificial erection is then carried out with normal saline (Fig. 6.1).
- The curvature is then assessed.
- The corpora is then denuded of the Bucks fascia till the albuginea is exposed sparing the neurovascular bundles.
- The opposite side of the curvature is then grasped with multiple Allis clamps so as to make the penis look straight (Fig. 6.2).
- Multiple inverting tunical inverting sutures with Prolene 4-0 sutures are taken till the curvature is corrected (Fig. 6.3).
- The penile skin is then repositioned and sutured back with Chromic catgut 3-0 and a light compressive dressing is placed.
- Catheter was kept for 24 hours and sexual abstinence was advised for a period of 2 months.

7 Priapism

INTRODUCTION

Priapism is erection that persists beyond or unrelated to sexual activity. It is of two types:

Low Flow

This is because of priapism due to lack of outflow leading to congestion of blood in corpora and subsequent decrease in arterial flow leading to ischemia. In this there is anoxia of smooth muscle component of corpora.

Priapism is an emergency. Any delay in the treatment will result in corporal ischemia and fibrosis. This will lead to permanent erectile dysfunction and penile deformity.

High Flow

This is due to trauma to perineum causing arteriovenous fistula and increased flow. This is not an emergency.

HISTORY

Detailed history regarding intracavernosal injection of vasoactive agents, hematological diseases, substance abuse, and perineal trauma should be taken. The duration and any accompanying pain should be inquired. Any past history of priapism should be inquired.

CLINICAL EXAMINATION

Very important to feel for any malignant induration (metastases causing priapism), bruit in perineum (trauma related high flow priapism). These obviously pinpoint to etiology and help in treatment.

INVESTIGATIONS

1. Duplex Doppler ultrasound to differentiate between low and high flow priapism. Duplex ultrasound will reveal low flow and constricted cavernosal artery, while in high flow, the flow will be turbulent indicative of arteriovenous fistula.

2. Cavernosal blood gas analysis (important) pH <7.25, pCO_2 >60, pO_2 >30 (low flow). The arterial blood gas picture is reverse in high flow variant. This is an important necessary tool because it definitively pinpoints the type of priapism. It involves aspiration of blood from the corpora and sending it to ABG analyser (usually present in ICU).

MANAGEMENT

Low Flow Variety

1. Hematological disorders—always hydrate the patient first.
2. If priapism less than 4 hours—intracavernosal injection of phenylephrine bolus 500 mg repeated after 5 minutes. Importantly patient's vitals should be kept on monitoring.
3. If priapism more than 4 hours—drain one corpora with 21 G scalp vein with aspiration to remove old anoxic blood and inject a bolus of phenylephrine (1 ml of phenylephrine with 19 ml normal saline mixture). The scalp vein should be clamped for 5 minutes. Repeat the procedure if there is no response (Fig. 7.1).
4. Alternatively drain the corpora with 20 G scalp vein passively and let the blood drain out on its own. Initially the drained blood is dark anoxic slowly once the smooth muscle component of the corpora recovers red blood oozes out and that is the end-point of the drainage (Fig. 7.2).

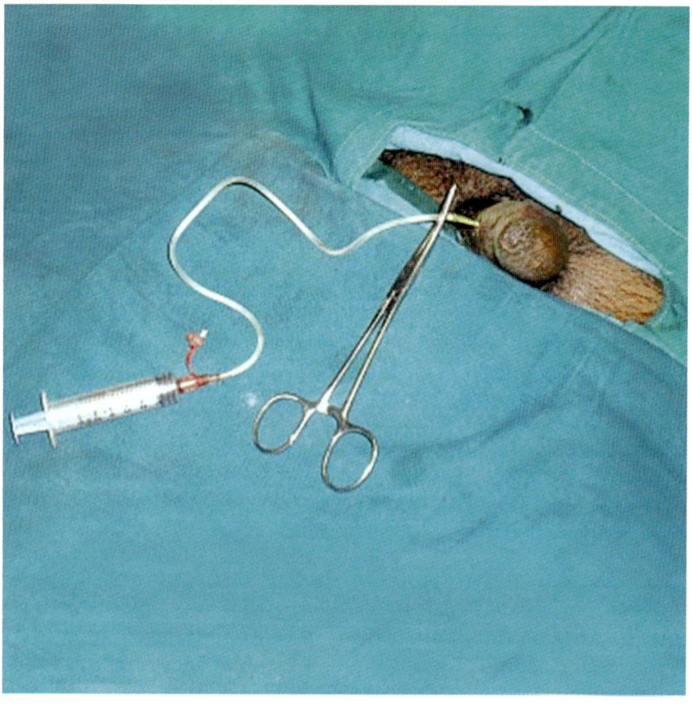

Figure 7.1: After injection of the phenylephrine the tube is clamped

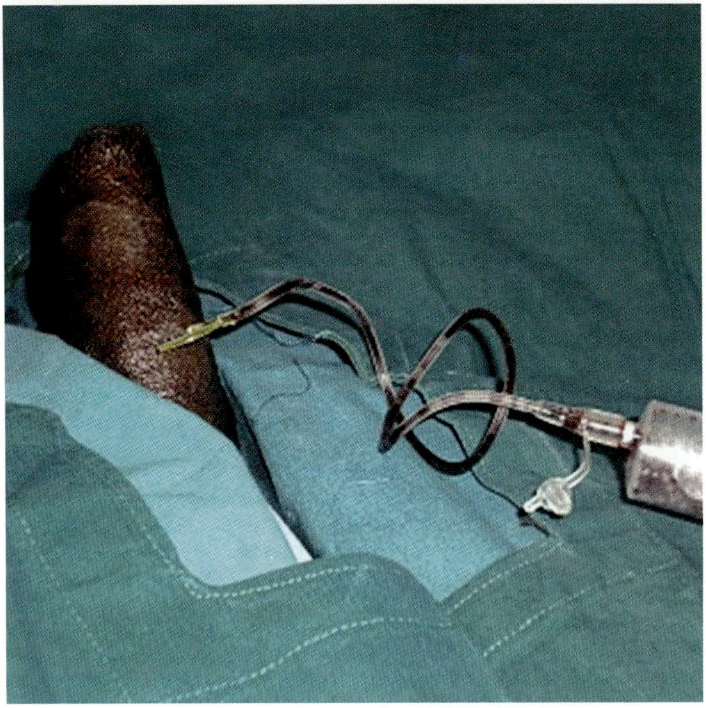

Figure 7.2: Dark anoxic blood being let out of the corpora

5. No response—send to andrologist for performance of corpora-glanular shunt (AL GHORAB SHUNT). This procedure is simple. It can be done under penile block anesthesia. It involves perforation of the corpora cavernosa through spongiosum (glans). This is followed by dilatation of the fenestration by Hegar's dilator. The aim is to allow drainage of anoxic cavernosal blood into relatively supple spongiosum. The glans wound is then closed. This procedure is safe and quick.

High Flow Variety

Initially conservative treatment like application of pressure-packing, ice-packing, use of adrenergic agents as written above. If these measures fail then internal pudendal angiography and angioembolization is the treatment.

STUTTERING PRIAPISM

Many patients, especially children, have a pattern of multiple short episodes over a period of days or several weeks. The priapism is often normal flow and prognosis is generally good and therapy is conservative. If the episode lasts longer and turns painful; then it should be like low flow variety. The long-term prevention can be done with Baclofen 40 mg at the bed time.

8 Penile Fracture

A penile fracture is an injury caused by the rupture of the *tunica albuginea*, which envelops the *corpus cavernosum penis*. It is most often caused by a blunt trauma to an erect penis.

PRESENTATION

A popping or cracking sound, significant pain, immediate flaccidity, and skin hematoma of various sizes are commonly associated with the event (Fig. 8.1). These symptoms are similar to a common bruising or contusion of the penis. If bucks fascia is intact then ecchymosis is confined to penis and the penis may appear like eggplant and if the bucks fascia is disrupted then "butterfly" hematoma may occur over the region of the perineum.

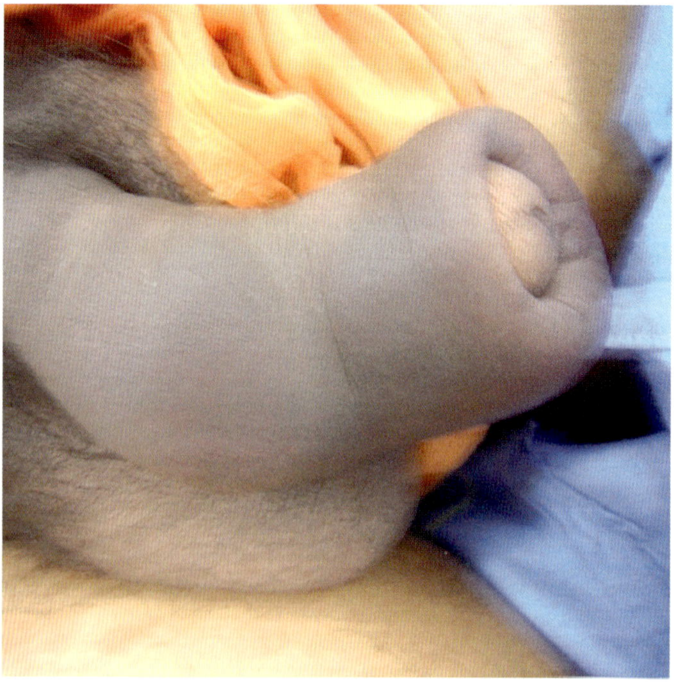

Figure 8.1: Penile fracture

CAUSES

In the western world the most common cause, accounting for about 30–50% of cases, is intercourse. Of those, woman-on-top position resulting in impact against the male pelvis or perineum and bending laterally are most common.

The practice of *taqaandan* also puts men at risk of penile fracture. Taqaandan, which comes from a Kurdish word meaning "to click," involves bending the top part of the erect penis, while holding the lower part of the shaft in place, until a click is heard and felt. Taqaandan is said to be painless and has been compared to cracking one's knuckles, but the practice of taqaandan has led to an increase in the prevalence of penile fractures in western Iran. Taqaandan is usually performed to achieve detumescence.

DIAGNOSIS

Penile fracture can be diagnosed by history or physical signs (a careful examination may reveal "Rolling sign"—palpation of blood clot over a break on tunica albuginea). In equivocal cases cavernosography or MRI may have to be performed. If urethral bleeding is also a presentation then retrograde urethrogram should be done to diagnose the urethral trauma.

TREATMENT AND PROGNOSIS

Penile fracture is a medical emergency, and emergency surgical repair is the usual treatment. Delay in seeking treatment increases the complication rate. Non-surgical approaches result in 10–50% complication rates including erectile dysfunction, permanent penile curvature, damage to the urethra and pain during sexual intercourse.

A circumferential degloving incision is given 1 cm proximal to the coronal sulcus then the trauma site is identified and the hematoma is evacuated. The defect in the tunica albuginea is repaired with inverting non-absorbable sutures.

9 Premature Ejaculation

Premature ejaculation (PE; also known as rapid ejaculation) is the most common type of sexual dysfunction in men younger than 40 years. Most professionals, who treat premature ejaculation, define this condition as the occurrence of ejaculation prior to the wishes of both sexual partners.

COMPLEX PROBLEM

Premature ejaculation sometimes is confused with delayed orgasm in female partner.

To explain, a male may reach climax after 5 minutes of sexual intercourse, but this is not premature ejaculation if his partner regularly climaxes in 3 minutes and both are satisfied with the timing. Another male might delay his ejaculation for a maximum of 30 minutes, yet he may consider this premature if his partner, even with foreplay, requires 45 minutes of stimulation before reaching climax.

Because many females are unable to reach climax at all with vaginal intercourse; they sometimes need foreplay simultaneously or before, this situation may actually represent delayed orgasm in the female partner rather than premature ejaculation in the male; the problem can be either or both, depending on the point of view. This highlights the importance of obtaining a thorough sexual history from the patient (and preferably from the couple).

HOW TO DEFINE PREMATURE EJACULATION?

The criteria for premature ejaculation stated in the *Diagnostic and Statistical Manual of Mental Disorders, Fourth Edition,* text revision *(DSM-IV-TR)* is as follows: (1) persistent and recurrent ejaculation with minimal sexual stimulation before, on, or shortly after penetration before the person wishes it; (2) marked distress or interpersonal difficulty; and (3) not exclusively due to direct effects.

CAUSATIVE FACTORS

This can either be primary since beginning or secondary after having period of normal ejaculatory latency. Many research articles are published regarding the causative factors for premature ejaculation, but at large it is attributed to psychological factor. These men have increased intravaginal ejaculatory latency time. Hyperexcitability many times are due to strict religious upbringing, sexual taboo in family and society, previous traumatic sexual experience and sexual abuse. Sometimes guilt of previous sexual exposure also contributes to the premature ejaculation.

Sometimes, performance anxiety plays important role in PE. The male often then gives excuse that the female partner excited him so much that he could not hold back.

Nowadays underlying erectile dysfunction also has been seen as cause for premature ejaculation.

Sometimes, cardiac patients ejaculate early having fear in mind that prolonged sexual act may precipitate heart attack.

MANAGEMENT

Many times detailed sexual history only suffices, no other investigations are really necessary.

Sexual counseling plays important role as to remove/allay previous fear/guilt from the minds of patients.

Step by Step Approach may Help Patients Many-a-times

1. Engaging in a lot of foreplay thus removing performance anxiety and avoiding actual insertional sex.
2. Squeeze-pause technique popularized by Masters and Johnson where partner masturbates the patient and before the climax, squeezes the glans (the pressure should be applied underneath the glans) to stop the ejaculate and ceases to stimulate the organ. Once the male organ is flaccid again, the female partner starts the technique again. This is repeated to gradually increase the ejaculatory latency.
3. After that female should stride across the male partner on his lap and repeat the same thing but only difference is that the penis is rubbed to the vulva *(no insertion again).*
4. Finally, they can engage in sexual act with the female partner on the top.
5. Once this sets the sex right, normal conventional position can be tried.

Drugs: Novel Drug, Dapoxetine in Premature Ejaculation

Normally selective serotonin uptake inhibitors are used for such patients along with psychotherapy. The mechanism of action of SSRIs is linked to their inhibition of neuronal uptake of serotonin in the CNS. Various animal studies suggest that SSRIs have weak effects on norepinephrine and dopamine neuronal reuptake. They prolong the sexual climax causing relief from early unwanted ejaculation.

These SSRI (Sertraline, Paroxetine, Fluoxetine) may take until at least 3 weeks following initiation of treatment to cause improvement in sexual latency.

It has been seen that many patients with PE have underlying erectile dysfunction also so adding PDE-5 inhibitors like Viagra (sildenafil), Tadalafil works well.

Dapoxetine is an SSRI developed specifically for the treatment of premature ejaculation. Dapoxetine may be effective at first dose (i.e. on-demand) for premature ejaculation when given 1–3 hours prior to sexual intercourse.

The optimal medical treatment for premature ejaculation has not been established but single dosing prior to sexual relations can work for many males. While raised blood levels through daily use of the medication may be unnecessary resulting in many CNS side effects. Obviously, if single dosing is successful, therapy is simpler and is associated with fewer adverse effects. Therefore, this may be the preferred initial therapy.

CERTAIN OTHER METHODS

Wearing condom, applying lignocaine jelly sometimes is practised. These agents may reduce penile sensitivity and excitability and delay ejaculation. Some andrologist give tramadol—centrally acting opioid drug (weak μ-opioid effect) in addition to reuptake inhibition of 5-HT and norepinephrine.

Circumcision practiced thinking that keratinization of the glans may help in reduction of sensitivity of the glans is occasionally practiced but it is a painful option with seemingly doubtful benefit.

Premature ejaculation in most cases is psychological. Sexual counseling of both partners is necessary (unlike in India, most of the times only male partner visits). The female partner's thinking it as *his problem rather than their problem.* SSRIs along with PDE-5 inhibitors in most cases along with Master and Johnson's technique are helpful. Condom and lignocaine jelly can complement for the delay in ejaculation.

10 Male Infertility

INTRODUCTION

Infertility is defined as the failure to conceive after one year of unprotected intercourse. The condition affects about 15% of couples within the reproductive age group and the male partner is contributory in about half the cases.

Basic clinical evaluation of the infertile male should include detailed reproductive history, physical examination and at least two semen samples must be obtained, preferably about a month apart with a 3–5 days abstinence period prior to each sample. According to abnormality in seminal parameters the following categories are made:

Oligo/astheno/teratospermia (OATs)

Abnormality in sperm density, motility or morphology. Updated reference values of sperm parameters by WHO in 2010 mentions.

- Quantity 1.5 ml
- Sperm concentration 15 millions/ml
- Progressive motility 32%
- Normal forms 4%

Sperm concentration and motility are the most important determinants for the need of Artificial Reproductive Technology (ART). Detailed has been mentioned regarding the management of asthenospermia in Flow chart 10.1.

Anejaculation

It is the inability to ejaculate despite of the stimulation. It can be psychological (anorgasmic), physical (orgasmic—due to ejaculatory duct obstruction/seminal vesicular pathologies or neurological) or situational (stress induced). Retrograde ejaculation occurs due to weakness of the bladder neck resulting in back flow of the semen in the bladder. Prostatic surgeries, medications like alpha blockers and neurological diseases can result in retrograde ejaculation. Vibrator therapy/electroejaculator treatment coupled with IUI can be used in such cases (Flow chart 10.2).

HORMONAL EVALUATION (FSH AND TESTOSTERONE)

An endocrine evaluation should be performed if:

1. Sperm concentration is less than 10 million/ml
2. Impaired sexual function such as decreased libido, volume of ejaculate.

Flow chart 10.1: Diagnostic algorithms in management of asthenospermia

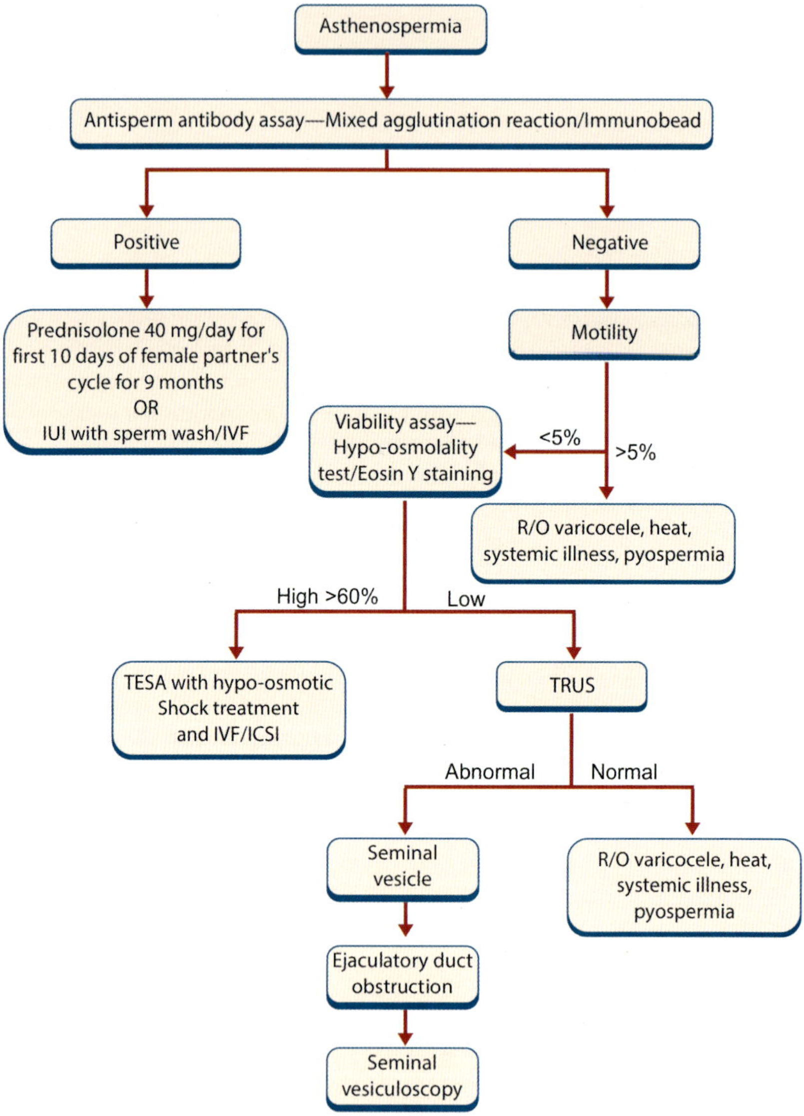

SEMEN CULTURE

Persistent pyospermia despite an initial course of empirical antibiotics is an indication for seminal culture. Cultures are often negative since the infecting organisms: *Chlamydia* and *Mycoplasma* cannot be grown on routine bacterial cultures.

Flow chart 10.2: Diagnostic algorithm in the management of anejaculation

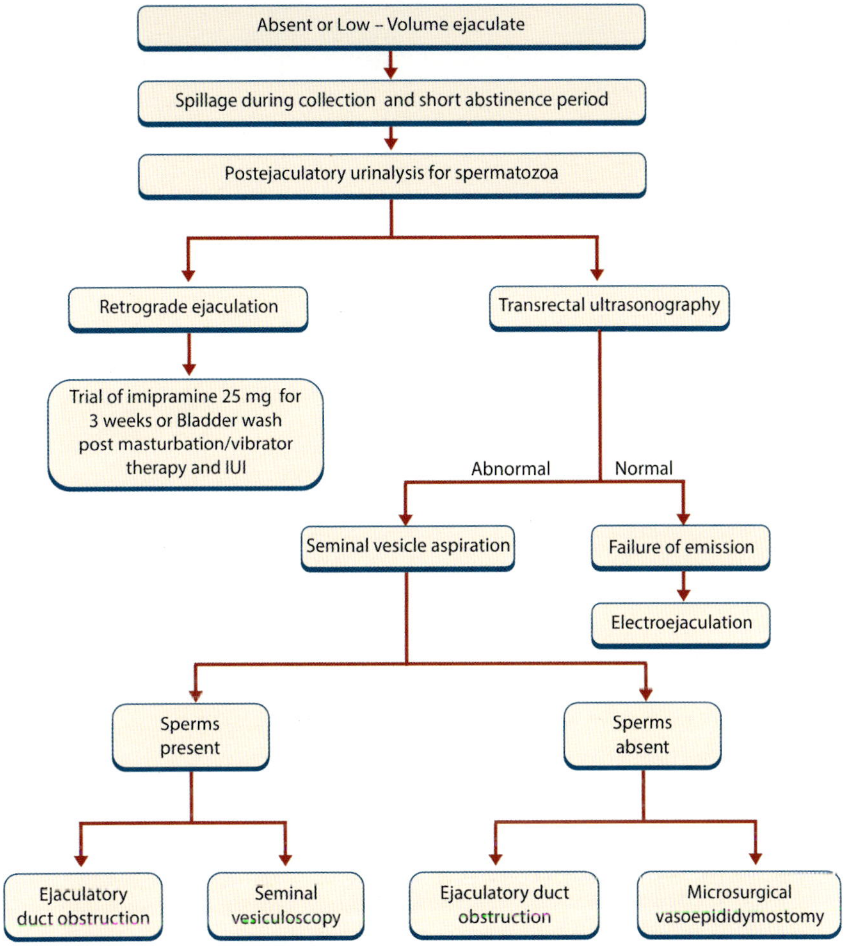

SCROTAL ULTRASOUND AND DOPPLER

Scrotal ultrasound should be done in case a suspicious mass lesion is found on clinical examination or the scrotum is difficult to evaluate clinically due to previous trauma/surgery/infection.

Varicocele can be reliable diagnosed with color Doppler ultrasound which shows dilatation of the pampiniform plexus more than 2.7 mm in diameter. Provocative maneuvers such as Valsalva maneuvers is asked to be performed to see the efflux (Figs 10.1A and B).

GENETIC TESTING

Genetic abnormalities may be present in up to 10% men with severe OATs. These are primarily deletions in the long arm of the Y chromosome (Yq microdeletions) or karyotypic abnormalities such as Klinefelter's syndrome or its variants. CFTR

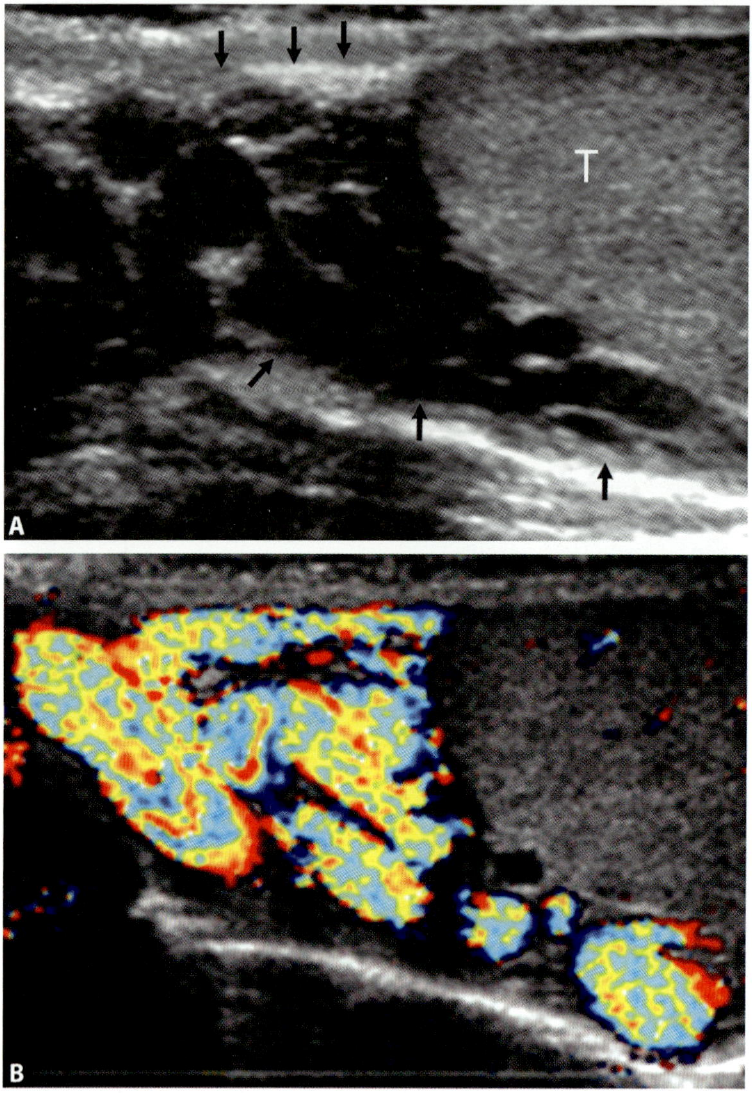

Figures 10.1A and B: Scrotal Doppler ultrasound showing dilated pampiniform plexus

gene testing is done in obstructive azoospermia with vasal agenesis. Detecting these abnormalities identifies the etiology of the infertility and allows counseling of the patients if they choose to undergo ART.

MANAGEMENT OPTIONS FOR OATs (NON-VARICOCELE RELATED)

Specific treatment must be offered to men with a demonstrable specific cause for OATs.

- Lifestyle changes, avoidance of heat exposure, toxin exposure should form the initial nondrug therapy for OATs.

- Hypogonadotropic hypogonadism requires hormone supplementation (Further details in topic of Pharmacology in Andrology).
- Pyospermia should be initially treated with a short course of agents effective against *Chlamydia* and *Mycoplasma*.
- Empiric therapies should be avoided in couples with advanced age or where the fertility potential of the female partner is compromised.
- There is no role of empirical androgens including testosterone, GnRH, FSH, hCG, hMG.
- Men with total asthenospermia with normal counts require ART.
- Sperm vitalisers and antioxidants can be used in idiopathic infertility (Idiopathic Oligoasthenoteratospermia) (Further details about these drugs in Pharmacology in Andrology Chapter).

INDICATIONS AND TECHNIQUES FOR CORRECTING A VARICOCELE

- A varicocelectomy should be advised only if all the following criteria are met:
  - Documented infertility
  - Clinically palpable varicocele
  - Presence of OATs
  - Fertile female partner.
- Adolescent boys with a demonstrably smaller ipsilateral testis or unmarried men with documented decline in semen parameters may also be counseled for a varicocelectomy.
- Azoospermic men with no other cause for azoospermia may rarely benefit from varicocelectomy, particularly if the varicocele is large or bilateral. Such men should be counseled well before surgery.
- Microsurgical procedures have the lowest risk of complications and should be preferred.
- Subinguinal approach is preferable as the pain is less because muscle cutting is not involved.

MICROSURGICAL VARICOCELECTOMY

- A 2 cm subinguinal incision is made
- With Babcocks forceps, the spermatic cord is held and brought out through the incision
- External spermatic vein is identified and ligated
- The cord is then placed over a Penrose drain
- With a magnification of 10–15; the surgery is started
- The external and internal spermatic fascia are opened longitudinally and retracted
- All the veins are dilated sparing testicular and cremasteric artery, vas, lymphatics and nerves (Fig. 10.2)
- Cremasteric box is closed.

The common complications like hydrocele, varicocele, varicocele recurrence, testicular artery injury are minimized by meticulous identification of structures in the cord with the use of magnification.

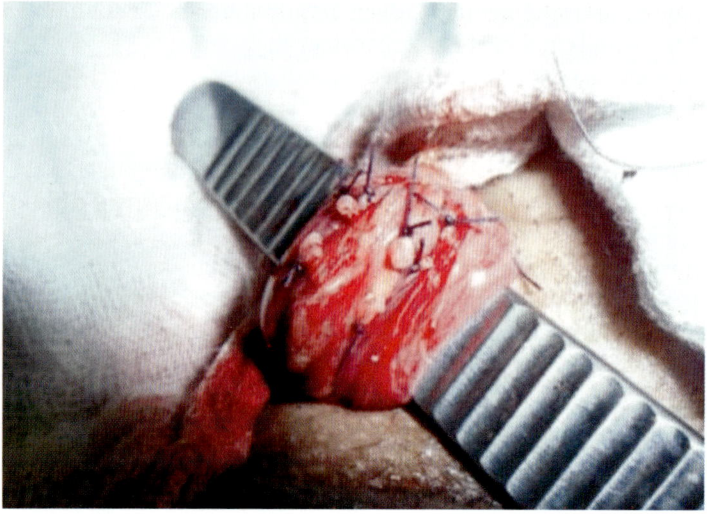

Figure 10.2: Varicocelectomy being performed under the loupe magnification

LAPAROSCOPY FOR VARICOCELECTOMY

Laparoscopy for varicocelectomy is challenging because of damage to testicular artery and higher recurrence rate however with the use of papaverine and meticulous dissection testicular artery can be preserved. This method can be probably used for bilateral varicocele (Table 10.1).

Azoospermia

Azoospermia refers to total absence of sperm. The presence of even a single mature sperm changes the diagnosis to extreme oligospermia or cryptozoospermia. Etiologies of azoospermia can be categorized into pretesticular, testicular and post-testicular. Pretesticular azoospermia occurs in men with hormonal

Table 10.1: Comparison of different techniques for varicocelectomy

Technique	*Artery preserved*	*Hydrocele (%)*	*Recurrence (%)*	*Potential for serious complication*
Microsurgical inguinal	Yes	0	1	no
Retroperitoneal	No	7	15–25	no
Conventional inguinal	No	3–30	5–15	no
Laparoscopic	Yes	12	5–15	yes
Balloon	Yes	0	7–25	yes

Goldstein, et al. Urology 1992

Flow chart 10.3: Diagnostic algorithm in the management of azoospermia

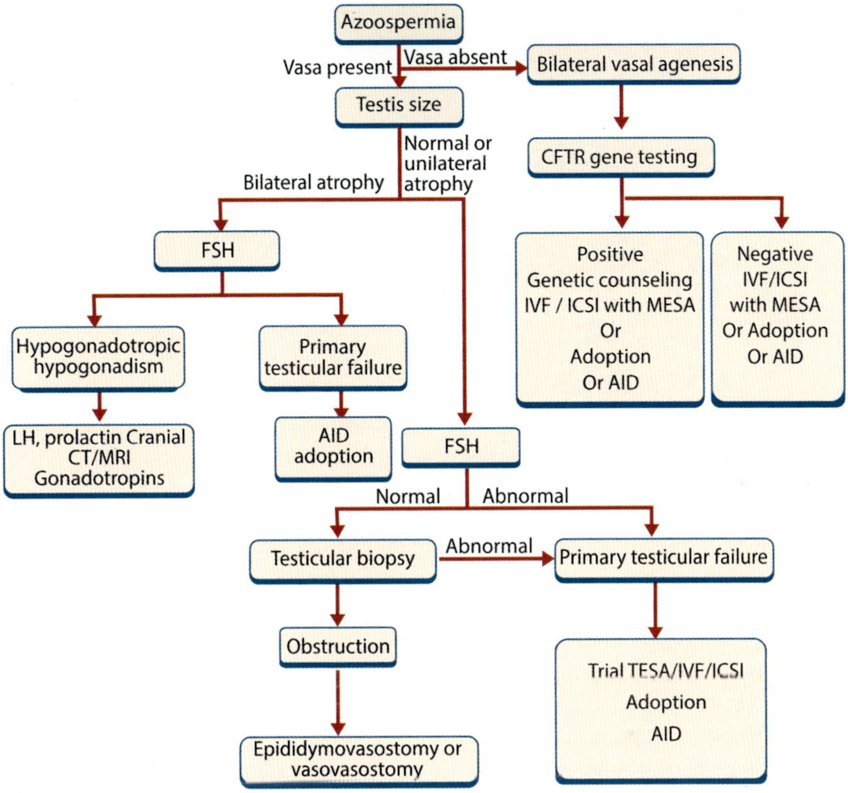

AID: Artificial insemination donor
TESA: Testicular sperm aspiration
MESA: Microsurgical epididymal aspiration

abnormalities and are uncommon. Testicular causes result in poor spermatogenesis. These are usually not amenable to corrective therapy and require ART. Post testicular causes are due to ductal obstruction or ejaculatory dysfunction. These are often correctable and the aim of evaluation of azoospermic men is primarily to identify such patients. Evaluation and management algorithm of azoospermia as given in Flow chart 10.3.

ADDITIONAL INVESTIGATIONS

Hormone Analysis

- Bilaterally small testis with FSH raised more than 2 × normal is diagnostic for testicular impairment and these men may not need a diagnostic testicular biopsy/FNAC.
- Serum FSH estimation is optional in men with obstructive azoospermia.

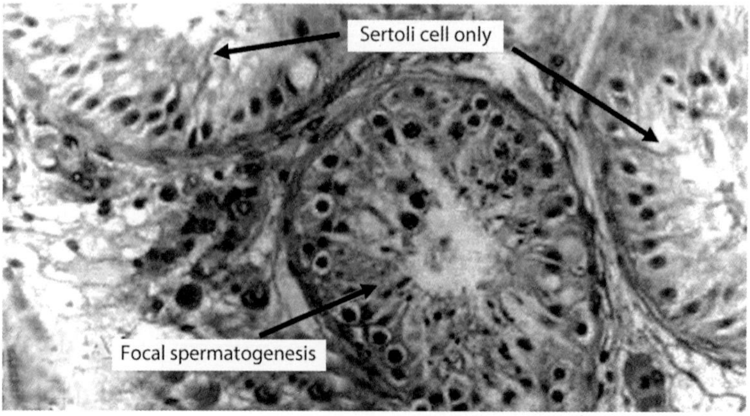

Figure 10.3: Testicular biopsy showing Sertoli cell only syndrome with focal spermatogenesis

Testicular Biopsy

- Testicular biopsy is mandatory before diagnosing obstructive azoospermia in men with a normal volume ejaculate and at least one palpable vas deferens.
- Testicular FNAC/needle biopsy provides diagnostic information as good as an open biopsy. Where feasible, FNAC/needle biopsy should be used instead of an open biopsy (Fig. 10.3).

Vasography

Vas patency may be confirmed by saline infusion or similar tests that do not result in inflammation of the vas. This should usually be combined with a reconstructive procedure and should not be performed as a separate diagnostic test.

Transrectal Ultrasonography (TRUS)

- TRUS is indicated in men with low-volume ejaculate and a palpable vas deferens.
- TRUS with injection of dye into the seminal vesicles is performed immediately prior to a transurethral resection of ejaculatory ducts (TURED) in men with ejaculatory duct obstruction.

Post-ejaculate Urine Examination

- Post-ejaculate urine should be checked for sperms in men with low-volume azoospermia, normal TRUS and normal spermatogenesis.
- Urine should be alkalinized for 2 days prior to the test.

Abdominal Ultrasound

Ultrasound of the abdomen, particularly the kidneys should be obtained in men with congenital bilateral absence of the vas deferens (CBAVD). These men have a higher incidence of renal agenesis.

DIAGNOSIS AND MANAGEMENT

Vasoepididymal Junction Obstruction (VEJO)

- Most cases of VEJO are idiopathic.
- Diagnosis is to be made if all the following are present:
  - At least one palpable vas deferens
  - Normal volume ejaculate with positive fructose
  - Normal spermatogenesis on FNAC
- Should be treated with a microsurgical vasoepididymal anastomosis
- The possible patency rates must be discussed with the patient before the surgery (30–50%).

Microsurgical Vasoepididymal Anastomosis

- We perform the surgery under spinal anesthesia
- High hemiscrotal incision is made
- The vas is isolated and transected at distal most site
- Proximal patency is checked with a saline vasogram (If saline goes freely; it indicates no proximal blockage)
- The vas tunica is then sutured to the tunica of the epididymis with distended tubules with Proline 8-0.
- The magnification used is 20–25
- We typically follow 2 suture intussusception technique described by Chan et al although some prefer three point intussusception technique (Fig. 10.4)

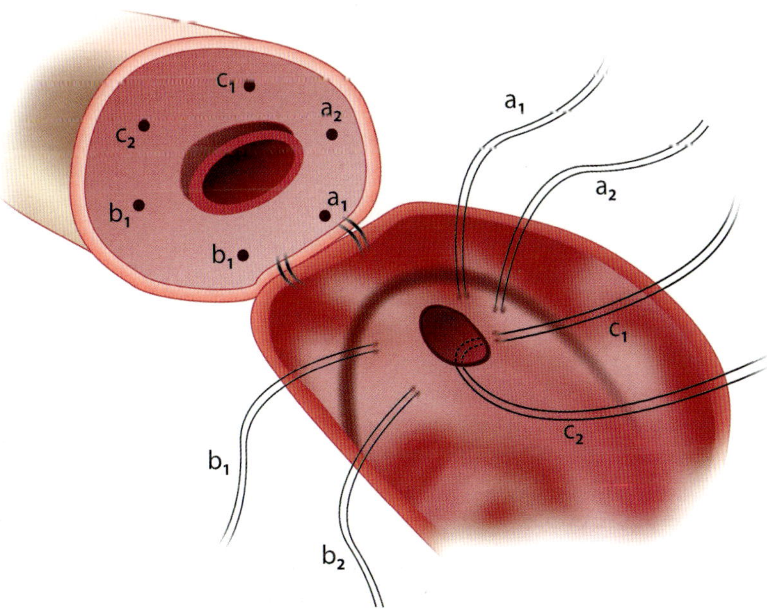

Figure 10.4: Three-point intussusception technique of vasoepididymostomy as described by Dr Brandell and Dr Goldstein

- Two double armed 10-0 Nylon sutures (Ethicon 3313) are placed longitudinally on a distended tubule
- The tubule is then punctured and fluid that oozes out is checked for sperms
- If sperms are present then we proceed further.
- If they are not present then we search for tubules on body or head of the epididymis
- The epididymal tubule is intussuscepted into the vasal lumen by 4-point fixation.
- The epididymal tunica is then sutured to the vasal tunica with 8-0 Proline.

Ejaculatory Duct Obstruction

- Diagnosis is to be made if all the following are present:
  - At least one palpable vas deferens
  - Low volume ejaculate
  - Absent of sperms on post-ejaculate urine examination
  - Normal spermatogenesis on FNAC testis
- Men with EDO and dilated ejaculatory ducts may benefit from transurethral resection of the ejaculatory ducts (TURED) or seminal vesiculoscopy.
- Results in the appearance of sperm in the ejaculate in about one-half to three-fourths of cases. The pregnancy rate achieved by this surgery is about 25 percent
- Retrograde ejaculation and recurrent urinary tract infections are complications usually encountered.
- Seminal vesiculoscopy liberally, safely deroofs seminal vesicles and bypasses the ejaculatory duct that too under direct vision. So the chance of restenosis is less likely.
  - Normal spermatogenesis on FNAC testis
  - Dilated seminal vesicles on Trans Rectal Ultrasound (TRUS) OR Pelvic MRI (Fig. 10.5).

Seminal Vesiculoscopy

- We use Richard Wolf 6/7.5 Fr ureteroscope and 10 W Revolix LASER for performing seminal vesiculoscopy
- The access is through the verumontanum (Trans-utricular) (Fig. 10.6)
- Once we enter the utricle then we fenestrate the utricle blindly superolaterally
- This area gives away easily without application of a force and we enter into the seminal vesicles
- We conclude the procedure by enlarging the seminal vesicular fenestration and deroofing the utricle with LASER (REVOLIX 10 W).

Vasectomy, Vasal Injury

- The diagnosis is usually evident from the history and examination.
- In patients with a long history of injury, spermatogenesis should be confirmed prior.

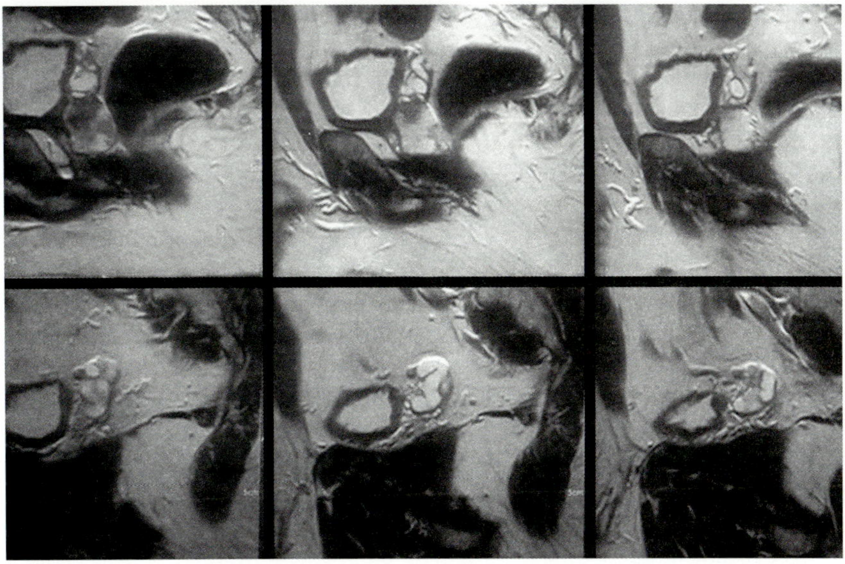

Figure 10.5: MRI showing seminal vesicular dilatation

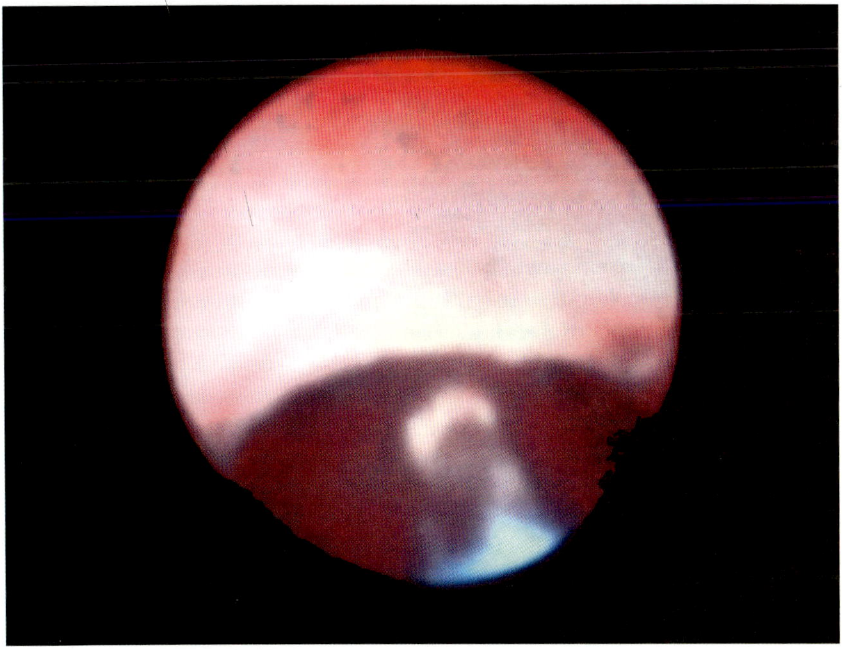

Figure 10.6: Seminal vesiculoscopy showing transutricular fenestration of seminal vesicles

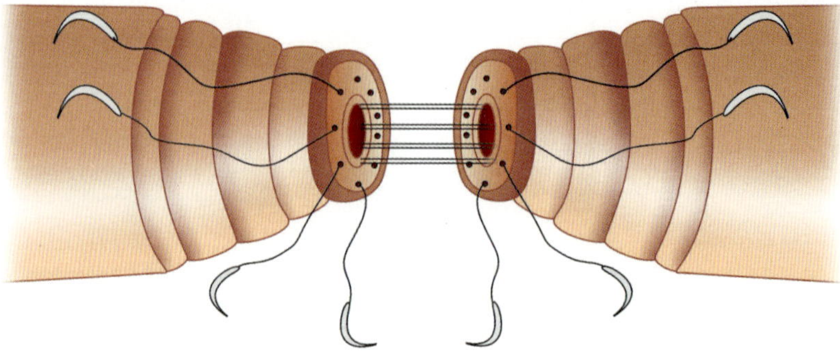

Figure 10.7: Microsurgical vasectomy reversal with Goldstein technique (Goldstein et al J Urol 1998)

- Microsurgical reconstruction treatment of choice (Fig. 10.7).
- The results in our setting is around 80–85% (patency rate).

TESTICULAR SPERM RETRIEVAL

1. For patients with nonobstructive azoospermia, recommend open testicular sperm extraction.
2. For cases of obstructive azoospermia, either open or percutaneous techniques may be used.

The Modalities of Sperm Extraction

Obstructive Azoospermia

Percutaneous epididymal sperm aspiration: The idea behind epididymal sperm acquisition is that higher yield of bankable sperms from the epididymis than the testis. As the percutaneous technique is unreliable the Microsurgical Epididymal Sperm Aspiration (MESA) has been method of choice for the sperm acquisition. It involves microsurgically exposing and incising epididymal tunic and aspirating epididymal fluid. MESA leads to extraction of large number of motile mature sperms which can be cryopreserved.

Non-obstructive azoospermia: Two methods have been described: Percutaneous (Fine needle aspiration or percutaneous aspiration with 14 G needle) or testicular biopsy. But the yield is scanty or none in Sertoli cell only syndrome or early maturation arrest. In these cases either random multiple biopsies or micro-dissection TESE have been employed with reasonable success rate. Microdissection technique employs inspection of individual seminiferous tubules under operating microscope and selecting opaque yellowish tubules and dissecting them out and examining them under microscope for spermatogenesis. The yield in this method more with very less testicular tissue damage.

ASSISTED REPRODUCTION

- Assisted reproduction should be the primary treatment modality in men with:
  - Testicular failure with severe OATs or azoospermia
  - CBAVD
  - All immotile sperms
  - Partners who have an indication for ART

11 Vasectomy

INTRODUCTION

It is a procedure where the vas deferens of a man is severed under local/sedative anesthesia so as to block passage of the sperms in the semen for the purpose of contraception.

HISTORY

The term vas deferens was coined by Berengarius (1470–1530). In Latin language, vas means vessel and deferre means 'to carry down'.

Vasectomy is a historical, social, philosophic, medical, demographic, and legal phenomenon. There have been constant attempts at renewing the techniques for simplicity and better outcomes. There are lot of misconceptions, false beliefs, and erroneous indications.

Early Years then in 1830, Sir Ashley Cooper's found that when the blood vessels of a dog's testicle were tied, no issues followed coitus. This was the first step towards development of a surgical procedure for birth control in men called vasectomy. The dog, however, retained its ability to produce sperms even after 6 years of the surgery.

The first use of vasectomy (1899) was on a 19-years-old male, who had complained of excessive masturbation. The surgery was carried out by a physician by name Harry Sharp. (? Logistics behind the surgery).

Between 1904 and 1907, vasectomy was used to reduce the chances of infection of the epididymis following prostate surgery.

The infamous case where a patient murdered a surgeon, for castration as birth control measure, prompted surgeons to look for another alternative for castration and very soon, vasectomy began to assume an important role.

The vasectomy became so fashionable that it was made compulsory of any confirmed idiot, rapist or a criminal. This led to the flourishment of the concept of eugenics where individuals, who were considered as being nuisance to the society, were vasectomized so ensure that the future generations were healthy?

VASECTOMY IN INDIA

The 1st vasectomy program on a national scale was launched in 1954 in India. In 1976, a huge government campaign for sterilization was launched and was responsible for the sterilization of millions of Indian couples. Health Ministry had then to face a lot of criticism for carrying out forced vasectomies of men and sterilization of women as a part of the initiative to control population.

Indications

- Contraception
- There are controversial indications for excessive masturbation and for social reasons as explained earlier.

Risks

A relationship between vasectomy and increased risk of prostate cancer was postulated (relative risk of 1.6) based on two large cohort studies. The magnitude of the relative risk is small enough to potentially be explained by the reason those patients who undergo vasectomy are usually people with more health awareness. So these people are more like to undergo prostate cancer screening than the general public.

Myths and Misconceptions

1. Vasectomized people do not ejaculate: *wrong.* More than 95% of the ejaculate comes from prostate and the seminal vesicles and only 3% is contributed by the testes so the ejaculate remains the same whether the patient gets vasectomized or not.
2. Men become less masculine. Testosterone continues to be produced even after vasectomy.

Benefits

Apart from contraception men are found to increase sexual quality of life probably because of decreased insecurity of making the partner pregnant.

Procedure

Usually done in an outpatient setting, a traditional vasectomy involves numbing (local anesthetic) of the scrotum after which small incisions are made on the hemiscrotum, allowing a surgeon to gain access to the vas deferens. The "vas" is cut and sealed by tying, stitching, cauterization (burning), double folding onto itself or burying in the scrotal fascia.

Modifications

1. *The No-Scalpel method:* Dr. Shunqiang developed the non-scalpel vasectomy popularized as NSV in 1974. It has less complication rate: pain, early recovery, no scar, etc. Over 15 million people have undergone NSV since 1974 and the number is increasing. In India this facility is made available by training the Primary Health Centre Officers so that even remotest place also people can undergo NSV. In this method a sharp hemostat, rather than a scalpel, is used to puncture the scrotum and by rotation bring the vas out. The vas is

then stripped and with any of the methods outlined above vasal severance can be carried out.

Country	*Number of NSV*	*Hematomas (%)*	*Infection (%)*
China	179,741	160 (0.09)	1,630 (0.91)
New York (USA)	238	0	0
Barcelona (Spain)	400	0	0
India	4,253	2 (0.047)	3 (0.07)

2. *No needle non scalpel vasectomy:* Wilson in 2001 initially described this technique. The jet technique of injection obviates use of the needle and has almost 100% efficacy rate.
3. *An "open-ended" vasectomy* obstructs only one end of the vas deferens, which allows continued pouring of sperm into the scrotum. This method may avoid build-up of pressure in the epididymis. Testicular congestion may also be reduced using this method.
4. *The "Vas-Clip" method* uses a clip to squeeze shut the flow of sperm. This method may facilitate a better outlook for reversal, as well as reduced pain with probably less success rate.
5. Percutaneous chemical vas occlusion (with silastomers) technique: with reportedly 98% success rate.

PREOPERATIVE COUNSELING

- This is a permanent method of contraception and reversal is technically challenging procedure.
- Regarding the procedure details and the possibility of hematoma and pain postoperatively.
- Those patients apprehensive can cryopreserve the sperms.
- The slight chance of failure (1:500 short term and 1:4500 long term) should be explained.
- Contraception is not immediate so for first few weeks he may have to use other methods for contraception (may need 6–8 weeks for azoospermia and about 20–25 ejaculations for the same).
- Patients with unstable relationship with the partner need to give a serious thought regarding the procedure.
- Patient needs to be emphasized that the vasectomy does not protect against STDs and HIV infection.
- Some men are forced by spouses to undergo the surgery in that case, the men should be totally convinced and satisfied for the reason.

Why female tubal ligations are more (worldwide 5 times more than the vasectomy) this is in spite the mortality rate of vasectomy is 0.1/1 lakh while that of tubal ligation is 4/1 lakh population)

1. Fear in men regarding the surgery

2. The tubal ligation can be combined with the cesarean section so it becomes convenient for the couple to go for it after they decide to complete the family.
3. Men forcing the female partner to undergo the procedure (India is a male dominated society).

COMPLICATIONS

Hematoma, bruising, local pains are some of the uncommon complications (0.1–3%) (Rather common with the conventional vasectomy not NSV).

Sperm granuloma: this can occur in 30% of the people because of the leakage of the sperms from the vasectomy end. *Chance of surgical recanalization is better in sperm granuloma because there is no back pressure blow-outs and secondary epididymal obstruction making reversal difficult.*

Postvasectomy Pain Syndrome

Postvasectomy pain syndrome (PVPS), genital pain of varying intensity that may last for a lifetime, (5% and 35% of vasectomized men), the pain can be orchialgia, pain during intercourse, ejaculation, or physical exertion, or tender testes. The pain usually may last for up to 3 months. In cases of persisting pain, several drugs like NSAIDs, tramadol, gabapantin have been tried with varied success.

In one study, vasectomy reversal was found to be effective for 9 out of 13 patients in reducing the symptoms of refractory chronic postvasectomy pain. Treatment options for the 4 patients, whose pain did not respond to vasectomy reversal were limited. *In severe cases castration has been resorted to.*

Postoperative Care

1. NSAIDs (pain killers) are given for pain relief.
2. Avoiding exertion and lying supine for 48 hours is recommended by many doctors.
3. Ice pack application can be resorted to, if the pain is refractory.
4. Sexual intercourse should be avoided for 1 week.
5. Patient should document absence of sperms at least on two occasions to prove that the procedure is successful before he relies totally on vasectomy for contraception.

Vasectomy Reversal

In 2–6% couples vasectomy reversal is undertaken either for desire to have children (change of the partner/change of mind to have more children/unfortunate loss of previous children, etc.). Some resort to it for unabating postvasectomy pain syndrome. This surgery is more successful (more than 80% results in our hands) done with microsurgical method. Earlier is the vasal recanalization better is the chance of success. (Success rate drops after 15 years of the vasectomy).

Vasectomy Reversal Procedure

- We use spinal anesthesia of vasectomy reversal
- High hemiscrotal incision is made

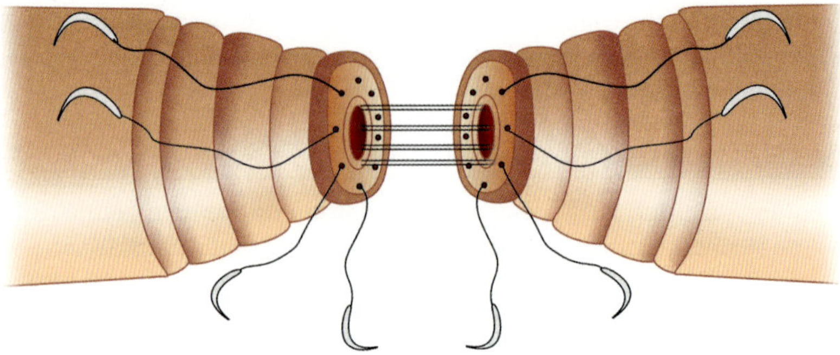

Figure 11.1: Microsurgical vasectomy reversal with Goldstein technique (Goldstein et al. J Urol 1998)

- Vas is isolated and cut sharply above and below previous vasectomy site
- Proximal patency is confirmed by saline vasogram
- The testicular end is compressed to squeeze fluid out through cut distal end of the vas
- As per the color, consistency and presence or absence of the sperms (sperms present and clear fluid—vasovasostomy/sperms absent/thick creamy fluid-vasoepididymostomy) further procedure is decided
- We use magnification power of 25
- Four sutures are taken at 12, 3, 6, 9 O' clock positions and mucosa to mucosa approximation is done (again 10-0 Nylon-Ethicon 3313 is used for the anastomosis) (Fig. 11.1)
- Four serosa to serosa approximating sutures are taken with 8-0 Proline.

FURTHER READING

1. Li S, Goldstein M, Zhu J, et al. The no-scalpel vasectomy. J Urol. 1991;145:341-4.
2. Viladoms JM, Li PS. Vasectomja sin Bistur. Arch Esp de Urol. 1994;47:695-701.
3. Liu X, Li S. Vasal sterilisation in China. Contraception. 1993;48(3):255-65.
4. V Kaza RM, Singh I, Singhal S, Kumaran V. An evaluation of the no-scalpel vasectomy technique. BJU Int (England). 1999;83(3):283-4.

12 New Innovations in Fields of Male Infertility

ROBOTS TO CURE MALE INFERTILITY

Recent studies have shown that male infertility is on the rise due to decrease in average sperm count, as we are step into the 21st century.

This can be attributed to genes, infections, lifestyle changes, smoking, drug abuse, mental stress due to pressures at work, obesity, hypertension, and environmental and pesticide pollutants. This means more and more males will become infertile and will have to resort to medical, surgical and assisted reproductive treatment to help their partners conceive.

Over the past 30 years, the treatment of infertility has seen the development of revolutionary new assisted reproduction techniques like in vitro fertilization (IVF) and intracytoplasmic sperm injection (ICSI).

These highly complex techniques are used with increasing frequency in the treatment of couples around the globe.

More than 1 million babies worldwide have been conceived by these new techniques giving immense satisfaction to infertile couples.

Both IVF and ICSI involve conception in a test tube and hence bypass natural conception. There is therefore a risk of undesirable genetic traits being passed on to next generation.

IVF and ICSI are also advised in males who have a poor sperm count and in whom medicine or surgery cannot help to improve the sperm count.

Recent technological advances have enabled the use of robotics and microsurgical assisted techniques to improve sperm counts. This helps conception in a more natural form and avoids the use of IVF and ICSI when the male is responsible for the lack of conception in an infertile couple.

The infertile males either have a low sperm count (due to inadequate sperm production also known as oligospermia) or have no sperms in the semen (Azoospermia).

When azoospermia is due to a block in the tubes (Epididymis, vas deferens, ejaculatory duct) transporting the sperm it can be cured surgically by advanced techniques called vasovasostomy, vasoepididymal anastomosis or seminal vesiculoscopy. These surgeries are very delicate and time consuming as they involve operating on structures smaller than the heart vessels.

With advances in microsurgery and robot assisted microsurgery, the chance of sperm (re)appearance rate can be as high as 80%. Without the use of these techniques the chances of sperm (re)appearance is as low as 5%.

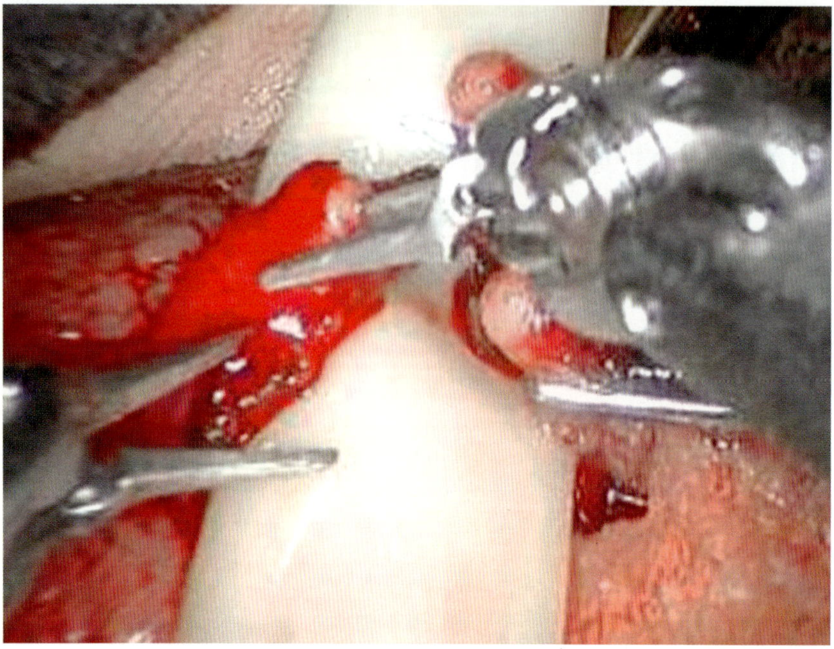

Figure 12.1: Dr Parekattil, University of Florida performing robotic vasectomy reversal

ROBOTIC VASECTOMY REVERSAL

It offers the microsurgeon an improved visualization, elimination of the tremor, decreased fatigue, greater freedom of motion and obviates the need for the skilled microsurgical assistant (Fig. 12.1).

The advantage of microsurgical reconstruction is that once successful, natural conception is possible time and again without the mental agony of going through multiple IVF or ICSI cycles apart from the huge recurring costs.

Multiple data from leading centers all over the world have proven the cost effectiveness of microsurgical and robotic microsurgical reconstruction over the routine sperm retrieval for IVF and ICSI.

In oligospermia (Low sperm count) due to poor sperm production either due to the enlarged veins surrounding the testes (varicocele), microsurgery allows a success rate of almost 60% (pregnancy rate).

In cases where the low sperm count is due to disease in the testes microsurgical sperm retrieval (Micro-dissection TESE) techniques can find sperm in testis.

In conclusion, recent advances in robotics and microsurgical techniques have given new hope to an infertile male to conceive in a natural way.

13 Andropause—Myth or Reality?

As a man ages, there is a gradual, progressive fall in total and free testosterone levels from age 30 onwards. With more and more senior citizens living longer, and seeking and demanding healthier, more fulfilling lives, the past decade has seen major advances in the perception and medical understanding of changes in physical, mental and emotional health of older men which were previously dismissed as 'normal aging'. It is now possible to distinguish normal age related decline in male hormone (androgen) levels from a clinical condition where a variety of physical, mental and sexual symptoms are caused by low androgen levels, and are thus eminently treatable by androgen replacement therapy.

PREVALENCE

Massachusetts male aging study: A prospective population base study in 1709 Caucasian men age 40–70 years at entry 7–10 years of follow-up showed that the total testosterone declined by 1.6% per year and the free testosterone declined by 2.8% per year. The albumin bound testosterone declined by 2.5% per year and sex hormone bound globulin (SHBG) increased by 1.3% per year. At age 60 years. Testosterone levels are decreased by 30–50%.

The medical community has however, and with good reason, been a bit guarded in recommending casual or nonspecialist diagnosis and treatment. This is because on the one hand the signs and symptoms are subtle and there are no straight forward diagnostic tests with clear-cut normal and abnormal values, and on the other hand treatment can have potentially serious side effects if used indiscriminately or without proper monitoring. Typical symptoms include decreased energy and chronic fatigue, sleep disturbances, mood changes and difficulty concentrating, and reduced sexual drive. Specialist evaluation will show signs of decreased muscle mass, decreased bone density, and increased visceral fat and hormonal abnormalities. All these symptoms can clearly also be due to other unrelated causes including financial and health related stress around retirement age, difficulty coping with changing relationships or death of a loved one, etc.—all major events which can start impacting one's quality of life at about the same time. Physical signs of androgen deficiency can similarly be mimicked by the tendency to put on weight in middle age, sedentary lifestyle, alcohol abuse and decreasing androgen levels due to something called the metabolic syndrome—a combination of inter-related disorders which increase the risk of heart disease, diabetes, etc. The main features of metabolic syndrome are putting on weight around the waist, high blood pressure, low 'good cholesterol' and tendency for diabetes.

MALE MENOPAUSE IS REALITY AND CAN SERIOUSLY COMPROMISE QUALITY OF LIFE

Recent research has shown that metabolic syndrome and age-related hypogonadism can be both cause and effect of each other. Therefore, the potential benefits of recognizing and treating 'male menopause' (or symptomatic late onset hypogonadism, to use the more accurate medical term) include not only improving the overall quality of life and sense of wellbeing, but also prevent more well-known killer diseases like heart disease, diabetes, blood pressure, etc. Hormone replacement will restore their lost manhood and thus improve sexual quality of life.

That is why experts the world over are coming to the consensus that in the presence of typical symptoms and documented hypogonadism, hormone replacement therapy is valid and effective. The androgen replacement therapy can cause increase in libido, improvement in erectile dysfunction, mood stabilization, increase in muscle mass, cognitive improvement and decreased incidence of fractures. There is also feeling of energeticness and improved glycemic control. There is also a cautionary note, however, because the diagnosis requires astute clinical judgement and treatment can have potentially serious side effects (like heart and liver dysfunction and the theoretical risk of prostate cancer), hormone replacement therapy should only be started after excluding any prostatic abnormality, and be carried out under specialist supervision and lifelong monitoring. Any concern about the prostate at any stage should warrant immediate urology referral. Male menopause is therefore very much a reality and can seriously compromise quality of life for ever-increasing numbers of men in their sunset years. But with very effective treatment available we all need to believe that getting old may be natural but feeling old is now optional.

14 Pharmacology in Andrology

MEDICAL MANAGEMENT OVERVIEW IN ANDROLOGY

Erectile Dysfunction

Pharmacotherapy of erectile dysfunction (ED could intervene in the CNS: Alpha 2 adrenergic blockers (Yohimbine, Phentolamine) and dopaminergic antagonist (Apomorphine) or peripherally agents that enhance, elevate or directly stimulates the synthesis of secondary messenger molecules such as cAMP or cGMP and direct activators of adenylate cyclase, for example, phosphodiesterase inhibitors: nonselective—papaverine, Type 5—sildenafil citrate, vardenafil, tadalafil, Type 3—milirinine and Type 4—rolipram.

Drugs for treating ED can be taken orally, injected directly into the penis, or inserted into the urethra at the tip of the penis. In March 1998, the Food and Drug Administration (FDA) approved Viagra, the first pill to treat ED. Since that time, vardenafil hydrochloride (Levitra) and tadalafil (Cialis) have also been approved. Additional oral medicines are being tested for safety and effectiveness. Viagra, Levitra, and Cialis all belong to a class of drugs called phosphodiesterase (PDE) inhibitors. Taken an hour before sexual activity, these drugs work by enhancing the effects of nitric oxide, a chemical that relaxes smooth muscles in the penis during sexual stimulation and allows increased blood flow.

While oral medicines improve the response to sexual stimulation, they do not trigger an automatic erection. The recommended dose for Viagra is 50 mg, and the physician may adjust this dose to 100 mg or 25 mg, depending on the patient. The recommended dose for tadalafil (Megalis, Forzest) is 10 mg, and the physician may adjust this dose to 20 mg if 10 mg is insufficient. A lower dose of 5 mg is available for patients who take other medicines or have conditions that may decrease the body's ability to use the drug.

None of these PDE inhibitors should be used more than once a day. Men who take nitrate-based drugs such as nitroglycerin for heart problems should not use either drug because the combination can cause a sudden drop in blood pressure. Also patients have severe cardiac diseases like recent myocardial Infarction; reduced stress tolerance should avoid PDE-5 inhibitors.

	Sildenafil	*Tadalafil*	*Vardenafil*
Maximum plasma concentration	30–120 (median 60)	30–360 (median 120)	30–120 (median 60)
Half-life hours	4	17. 5	4-5
Duration of action	up to 4–12	up to 36	Up to 4–12
Food restriction	May take longer to work with meals	Can be taken with or without food	Can be taken with or without fatty foods

INTRACAVERNOSAL INJECTION OF VASOACTIVE DRUGS (ICIVAD)

Many men achieve stronger erections by injecting drugs into the penis, causing it to become engorged with blood. Drugs such as papaverine hydrochloride (15-60 mg), phentolamine, and alprostadil (marketed as Caverject) widen blood vessels. These drugs may create unwanted side effects, however, including pain (36%) persistent erection (4%) and scarring. It gives a success rate of 70-90% but these injections have a drop-out rate of 25-60% because of mainly pain or sometimes development of corporal fibrosis.

Methodology of Giving Papaverine/Bimix

Start with 29-30 G Insulin syringe for the injection therapy.

Papaverine: It can be started with 15 and given till 60 mg. Inject in any corpus.

Bimix: Add chlorpromazine (4 ml papaverine to 0.1 ml chlorpromazine combination) start with 0.1 to 0.2 ml and then gradually increased. Again the injection can be given in any one of the corpus.

Drug Therapy for Peyronie's Disease

Medical Treatments

Various medications like vitamin E 400 mg three times a day for 3 months, Colchicine 0.5 mg 2 BD for 3 months or Tamoxifen 20 mg BD for 3 months. The placebo controlled trials have not shown efficacy of the medications but colchicines there are no placebo studies. It seems to be effective.

Researchers have also tried injecting chemical agents such as verapamil, collagenase, steroids, and interferon alpha-2b directly into the plaques. Verapamil and interferon alpha-2b seem to diminish curvature of the penis. The other injectable agent, collagenase, is undergoing clinical trial and results are not yet available. Steroids like triamcinolone have caused loss and atrophy of the local tissues and weakening of the tunica. The surgical planes also become difficult after steroid injection.

The intralesional injections are given with 24 G needle making multiple passes through the plaque. There is a possibility that the multiple passes make the plaque weak by mechanical disruption.

Intralesional Therapy

Intralesional Verapamil

- Dose 10 mg verapamil/4 ml + 6 ml saline total 10 ml; 2 weekly for 12 injections
- Promising but unproven.

Intralesional Interferon-alpha-2b

- Dose: 1 millon units 2 weekly for 12 injections
- Placebo trial-ongoing
- Possibly useful.

Intralesional Steroids

- Dose 40 mg triamcinolone/ml; dilute as per size 6 weeks total 6 injections
- Steroids may weaken tunica loss of surgical planes due to trauma.

IDIOPATHIC OLIGOSPERMIA: MANAGEMENT

Despite advances in diagnostic modalities up to 25% patients exhibits unexplained infertility. A variety of medical therapies have been suggested to treat this group. However, none of these have shown effective to be repeated controlled trials. A meta-analysis of all controlled studies for idiopathic male infertility has failed to reveal significant efficacy of currently available treatment. In the hope that they may be effective in a selective group of people a minimum of 3–6 months trial should be given to include at least one cycle of spermatogenesis.

The empirical therapy includes the following drugs:

1. *Hormonal agents (direct or rebound effect):* The testosterone undecanoate 80–160 mg/d, testosterone enanthate or propionate injection. Two to three weekly side effects: Azoospermia, gynecomastia, cholestasis and hepatic dysfunction.
2. *Antiestrogens:* Clomiphene citrate 25–50 mg daily, tamoxifen 10–30 mg daily, side effects: Nausea, weight gain, loss of libido, headache, gynecomastia, and dermatitis.
3. *Antioxidants:* The oligospermia is many times attributed to reactive oxygen species. Various agents are prescribed to nullify the effects of reactive oxygen species like glutathione, lycopene 4 mg/d, vitamin E 400–800 mg/d, N-acetyl cysteine 1000 mg/day.
4. *Sperm vitalizers:* Cellular energizers like L-arginine, zinc, selenium, proanthrocyanidin, carnitine 1–2 mg/d CoQ10 10–400 mg/d, pentoxiphylene.

If this is unsuccessful, assisted reproductive technique (ART) is employed or a combined approach may be started simultaneously in older couples.

SPECIFIC MEDICAL THERAPY IN OLIGOSPERMIA

Chronic Fungal Dermatitis

Antifungal topical cream, for example, Candid B ointment locally.

Chronic Filarial Epididymo-orchitis

Antifilarial and anti-inflammatory drugs—Hetrazan 100 mg three times a day for 3 weeks.

Seminal Infections

Whether infection causes infertility is still controversial. There are several conflicting reports of benefit of treatment. The semen analysis showing plenty of pus cells should be discussed with the seminologist so as to remove any confusion of round cells with immature spermatogonia. Semen culture should be done in such cases. The common seminal organisms are: *Streptococcus* fecalis, *E. coli,* coagulase +ve staph (albus) or occasionally *Klebsilla,* Proteus, *Pseudomonas.* Ciprofloxacin/doxycyclines can be administered as per the semen culture sensitivity report for a period of 4–6 weeks. As a rule, both sexual partners should be treated at the same time. In the meantime condom intercourse can be performed. At the end of the treatment it should be confirmed that infection is eradicated as there is tendency for chronicity.

Antisperm Antibodies

The direct test should be done for ASA and if present should be treated on priority with intrauterine insemination. The other modality of treatment is giving prednisolone 5 mg three times a day for 3–12 months.

Management of Hypogonadotropic Hypogonadism

Management of Delayed Puberty

No initiation of puberty by age 13 in girls and 14 in boys.

Delayed Puberty Management

Injection testosterone esters are given in the strength of 50–100 mg per month for 3–6 months. This dose will advance puberty without impairing height potential. The spontaneous onset of puberty should be awaited for 3–6 months if there is no initiation formal testosterone replacement therapy should be given.

Management of Prepubertal Hypogonadotropic Hypogonadism

The treatment should be based on androgenizing the patient. So, it is usually done by giving testosterone or hCG.

TESTOSTERONE REPLACEMENT THERAPY FOR ANDROGENIZATION

Injection sustanon deep IM in the following protocol: to start with 100 mg deep intramuscular every month for 3 months. This dosage is progressively increased to 250 mg once a month followed by 250 three weekly for long term treatment. When fertility is desired LH and FSH support is usually given with proper counseling as the cost of the therapy may be 2–3 lakhs with 50% chance of conception.

The underlying principle is to achieve initial testicular growth with LH (LH is given as hCG). 5000 u one injection per week, 2000 u two to three injections per week. hCG dose monitoring is done by assaying testosterone on day 3 (for response) and day 7 (for sustenance). Testicular volume is monitored along with the signs of androgenisation. When testicular volume become 18 ml and ejaculation starts then FSH are added to complete spermatogenesis. FSH is started in the form of HMG (Dose options: 37.5 units thrice-a-week/75 u thrice-a-week/150 u thrice-a-week).

This is continued till pregnancies occur. The count may increase from azoospermia to 5–10 millions/ml so assisted reproductive technology may be needed. Testosterone is restarted after pregnancy is over.

DRUGS THERAPY IN PREMATURE EJACULATION

Local Anesthesia

Topical anesthetics/gel is sometimes given with the idea of desensitizing the glans and delaying the orgasm. Lignocaine cream can be given for application for 20 minutes before the sexual act.

Medications

Normally selective serotonin uptake inhibitors are used for such patients along with psychotherapy. The mechanism of action of SSRIs is linked to their inhibition of neuronal uptake of serotonin in the CNS. They prolong the sexual climax causing relief from early unwanted ejaculation.

These SSRI (Sertraline, Paroxetine, Fluoxetin) may take until at least 3 weeks following initiation of treatment to cause improvement in sexual latency.

Dose of the Medications

- Clomipramine (clonil) 10–25 mg
- Paroxetine (parotin) 10–20 mg
- Sertraline (sertima) 25–100 mg
- Fluoxetine (prodep) 20–40 mg

These drugs may cause side effects like yawning, anejaculation, decreased libido, perspiration and increased fatigue.

It has been seen that many patients with PE have underlying erectile dysfunction also so adding PDE-5 inhibitors like viagra (sildenafil), tadalafil works well.

Dapoxetine is an SSRI developed specifically for the treatment of premature ejaculation. Dapoxetine may be effective at first dose (i.e. on-demand) for premature ejaculation when given 1–3 hours prior to sexual intercourse.

The optimal medical treatment for premature ejaculation has not been established but single dosing prior to sexual relations can work for many males. While raised blood levels through daily use of the medication may be unnecessary resulting in many CNS side effects. Obviously, if single dosing is successful, therapy is simpler and is associated with fewer adverse effects. Therefore, this may be the preferred initial therapy.

15 Setting up an Andrology Suite

Andrology literally means the science dealing with male sex especially male reproductive science.

MALE IMPOTENCE

The andrology clinic for evaluation of male sex organ usually does not need costly equipment. Routinely impotence can be evaluated by thorough medical, sexual and psychosexual history.

The sexual history can be aided by 5 points the International Index of Erectile Function. The five options for each question is from almost always to never.

Over the past 6 months					
1. How do you rate your confidence that you could get and keep an erection?	Very low	Low	Moderate	High	Very high
2. When you had erections with sexual stimulation, how often were your erections hard enough for penetration?	Almost never/ never	A few times	Sometimes	Most times	Almost always/ always
3. During sexual intercourse, how often were you able to maintain your erection after you had penetrated your partner?	Almost never/ never	A few times	Sometimes	Most times	Almost always/ always
4. During sexual intercourse, how difficult was it to maintain your erection to completion of intercourse?	Extremely difficult	Very difficult	Difficult	Slightly difficult	Not difficult
5. When you attempted sexual intercourse, how often was it satisfactory for you?	Almost never/ never	A few times	Sometimes	Most times	Almost always/ always

IIEF-5 scoring: The IIEF-5 score is the sum of the ordinal responses to the 5 items.
22–25: No erectile dysfunction
17–21: Mild erectile dysfunction
12–16: Mild to moderate erectile dysfunction
8–11: Moderate erectile dysfunction
5–7: Severe erectile dysfunction

The presence of laboratory that can perform fasting glucose, lipids, and hormonal profiles tests. These tests are performed primarily to identify or confirm specific causes (e.g. hypogonadism) or to assess the role of medical co-morbidities or concomitant illnesses (e.g. diabetes, hyperlipidemia).

All the patients with impotence can be started with phospho-diesterase inhibitors except for few patients on nitrates, low BP <90/60 mm Hg, active coronary artery disease, etc.

While energy expenditures during sexual intercourse may vary depending on many individual factors, estimates were obtained in a laboratory setting by Bohlen et al (1984) using the metabolic equivalent of energy expenditure (MET) in the resting state (equal to 3.5 ml/kg/min oxygen consumption) as a quantitative parameter. Healthy males attained 2.5–3.3 METs during sexual stimulation and orgasm with some variability (2.0–5.4 METs). For comparison with daily life activities, one might say that 3 METs equals briskly climbing two flights of stairs, and 5 METs may be compared with digging in the garden. A possible conclusion derived from these measurements might be that a patient, who is able to achieve 5–6 METs on exercise testing without signs of ischemia, major arrhythmia or inadequate increase of blood pressure, may not be at excess risk for a cardiac event during sexual activity. So by detailed clinical history such patient can be safely started with PDE-5 inhibitors.

Those patients who are not benefitted by medications can be started on intracavernosal injections. (As outlined before in previous chapter).

The patient can also be given option of vacuum erection device (Fig. 15.1).

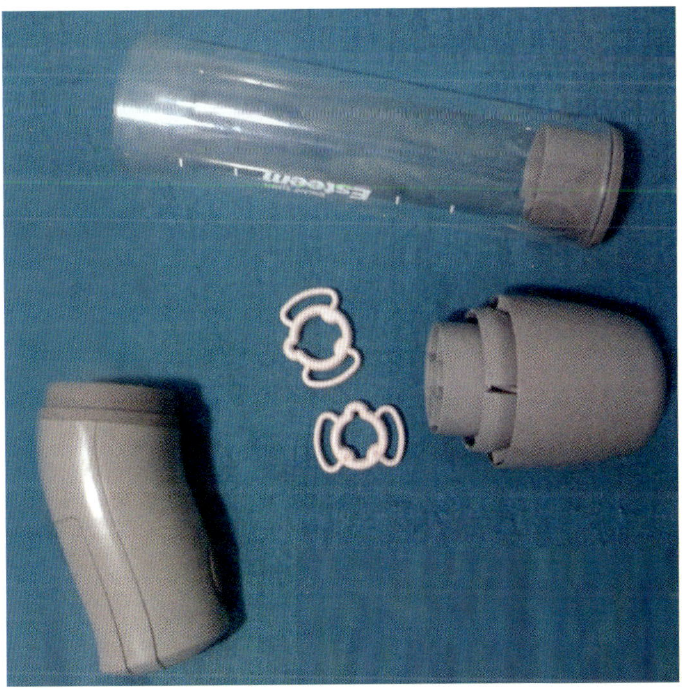

Figure 15.1: Vacuum erection device

Many of patients who find its use easy and it has allowed many couples to successfully resume penetrative sexual relations. A number of reports have cited satisfaction rates above 80%. This treatment has been shown to result in definite improvement in erection hardness, increase in frequency of sex and increase in overall sexual satisfaction. Increased satisfaction for the partner has also been demonstrated. Drop-out rates of up to 30% have been cited and the most common reasons for drop-out include inadequate rigidity, penile pain, failure to ejaculate and dissatisfaction with penile appearance and temperature. The vacuum device is suitable for all groups of patients with ED.

Some patients can be put on intracavernosal injections. Intracavernosal injections provide an effective therapy for men with erectile dysfunction who cannot take oral agents or for whom oral agents are not effective.

Basically, I would consider a patient not responding to these above said measures a complex one and go ahead with pharmacopenile Doppler test/ NPTR/angiography test. So basic andrology setup can be done with only few devices-vacuum erection devices, availability of papaverine/chlorpromazine mixture and insulin syringes, charts to take down IIEF scores, vibrators for aiding ejaculation. The clinician can decide for going for ultrasound Doppler machine/ NPTR-Rigiscan machine once the scope of his practice expands.

COLOR-DOPPLER ULTRASOUND

When vascular evaluation is indicated, intracavernous injection with color duplex Doppler ultrasound is the most informative diagnostic test (Fig. 15.2).

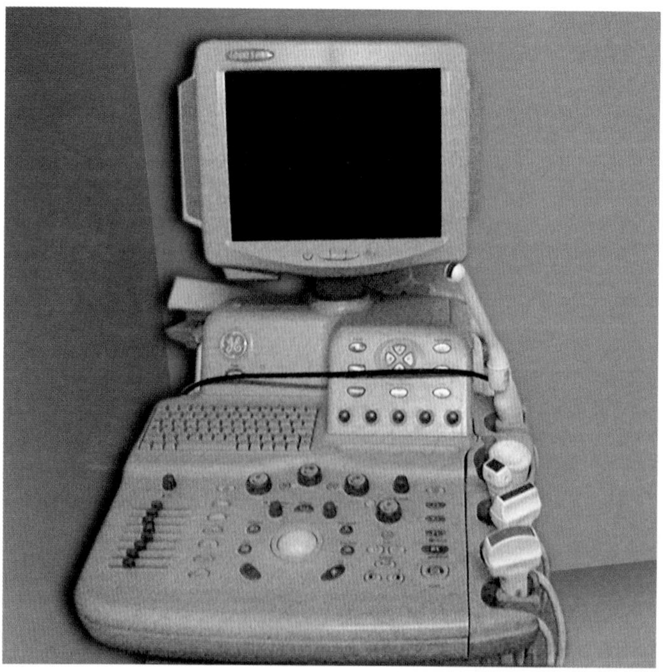

Figure 15.2: Color-Doppler ultrasound

This may be all that is needed to define and determine severity. Color duplex ultrasound should be used before other tests are considered because it is the least invasive technology for evaluating vascular ED, distinguishing high-from low-flow priapism, and assessing Peyronie's plaque. The parameters used to infer the integrity of the penile inflow tract are cavernous arterial diameters, peak systolic arterial velocity (PSV is the maximum of the systolic waveform), end-diastolic arterial velocity (EDV), systolic rise time (measured in msec from the start of systole to maximum value), cavernosal artery acceleration time (AT; PSV ÷ systolic rise time), and index of vascular resistance (RI; PSV-EDV ÷ PSV). PSV less than 25 cm/s after intracavernous injection and sexual stimulation has a 100% sensitivity and 95% specificity in selecting patients with abnormal penile arteriography, because it reflects severe cavernous arterial insufficiency. A PSV consistently greater than 35 cm/s is associated with normal arteriography and defines normal cavernous arterial inflow. Color duplex ultrasound accurately assesses venogenic ED (EDV> 5 cm/sec predicts venogenic impotence).

NOCTURNAL PENILE TUMESCENCE RIGIDITY TEST

In its classic form, NPT consists of nocturnal monitoring devices that measure the number of episodes, tumescence, maximal penile rigidity, and duration of nocturnal erections. In 1985, the RigiScan was introduced; it was the first device to provide automated, portable NPTR recording. The device combines the monitoring of radial rigidity, tumescence, number, and duration of erectile events with the convenience of a portable system that can be used at home. It consists of a recording unit that can collect data for three separate nights for a maximum of 10 hours each night (Fig. 15.3). The mechanics consist of two loops:

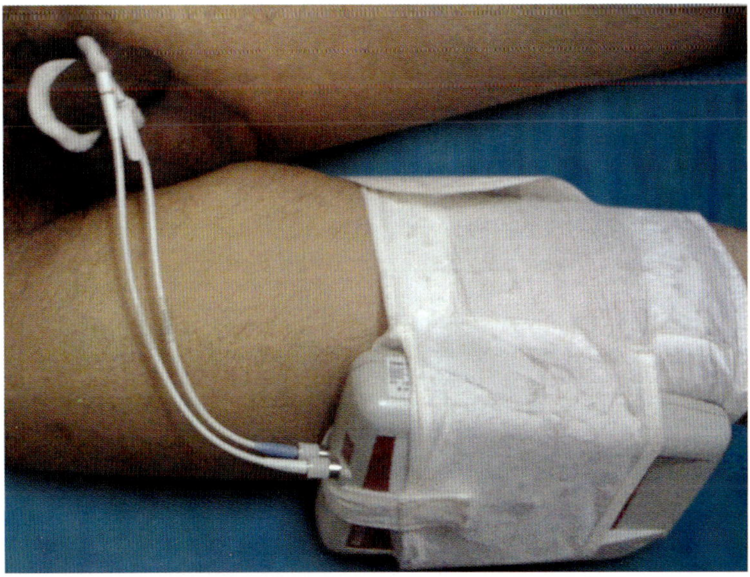

Figure 15.3: Penile tumescence rigidity test

one is placed at the base of the penis and the other at the coronal sulcus. By constricting the loops, the device records penile tumescence (circumference) and radial rigidity at the penile base and tip. Radial rigidity above 70% represents a nonbuckling erection, and a rigidity of less than 40% represents a flaccid penis. The number of erections considered normal is three to six per 8-hour session, lasting an average of 10 to 15 minutes each. The normal **NPTR** criteria are: four to five erectile episodes per night; mean duration longer than 30 minutes; an increase in circumference of more than 3 cm at the base and more than 2 cm at the tip; and maximal rigidity above 70% at both base and tip.

The documented presence of a full erection indicates that the neurovascular axis is functionally intact and that the cause of the ED is most likely psychogenic.

MALE INFERTILITY SET UP

All infertility setup should have facility for semen analysis. Clean, wide-mouthed containers should be used for specimen collection. Masturbation/Inert condoms/ coitus interuptus can be used to collect the semen and 4–7 days of the abstinence should be followed. In most cases, two or three specimens examined over a period of several weeks will give an adequate assessment of baseline spermatogenesis.

The World Health Organization defines the following reference values (WHO, 2000):

1. Volume: 1.50 ml or more
2. pH: 7.2 or more
3. Sperm concentration: 15×10^6 or more spermatozoa/ml
4. Motility: 32% progressive motility
5. Morphology: 4% or more by strict criteria

Semen analysis can be done after centrifugation with microscopy; Computer assisted semen analysis apparatus is not needed for semen analysis for management of the infertility.

Special tests: Anti-sperm antibody tests, quantitative fructose estimation in semen, specialize sperm viability tests can be performed at referral labs as these tests are not needed routinely.

Hormonal evaluation/genetic testing-chromatin or AZF testing also can be performed at referral lab.

Every andrologist should be able to perform trans-rectal ultrasound for seminal vesicular visualization and diagnose ejaculatory duct obstructions (Fig. 15.4).

For varicocele diagnosis usually clinical examination suffices but sometimes handheld Doppler can be used to diagnose the reflux in obese patients or previously operated groins (Fig. 15.5).

SURGICAL MICROSCOPE

The andrological reconstructive surgery needs good magnification and resolution so a microscope is a must thing for the set-up (Fig. 15.6). Microsurgical varicocelectomy needs a magnification from 10–15 × while vasoepididymostomies need a magnification of 25–30 ×.

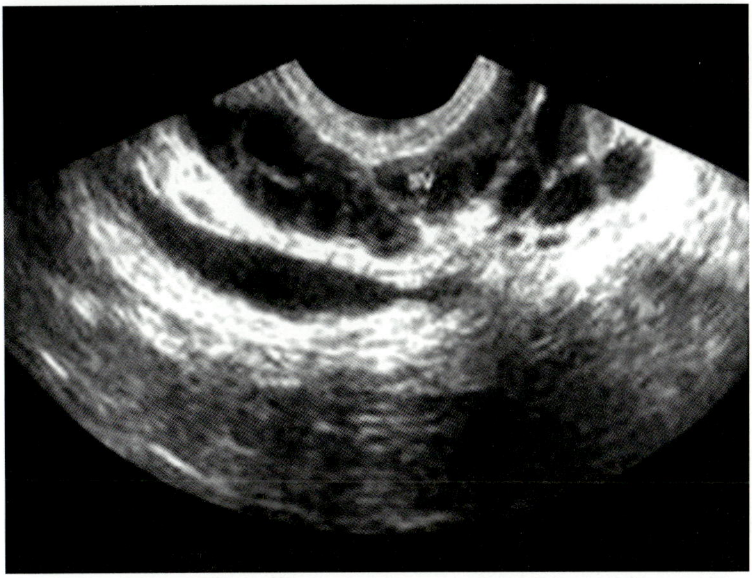

Figure 15.4: Ultrasound for seminal vesicular visualization

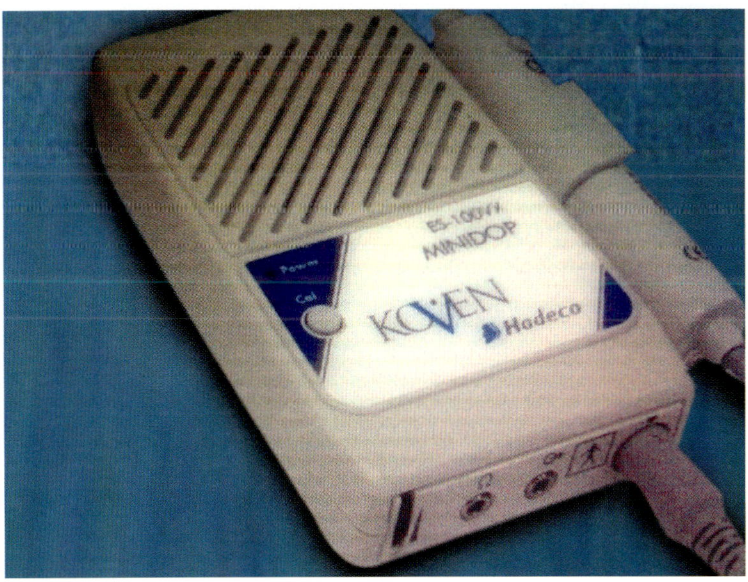

Figure 15.5: Handheld Doppler

To complete the set-up requirements—for hypogonadism in children—Praders orchidometer is an essential requirement to monitor gonadal growth/or to observe catch up growth phenomenon after varicocele surgery in adolescents.

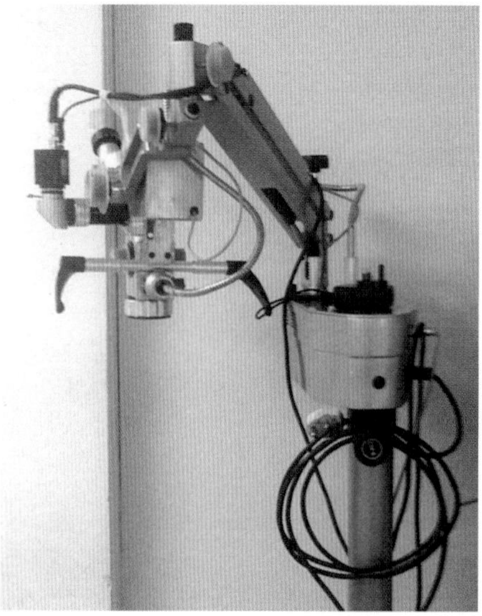

Figure 15.6: Surgical microscope

SPERM RETRIEVAL

Andrologist plays a pivotal role in diagnostic and therapeutic testicular biopsy. We usually prefer testicular biopsy with 14 G biopsy gun under cord block for diagnostic testicular biopsy as well as sperm retrieval in non-obstructive azoospermia. Only difference in non-obstructive azoospermia multiple biopsies may be needed to tackle the problems with patchy spermatogenesis.

For obstructive azoospermia either MESA (**M**icrosurgical **E**pididymal **S**perm **A**spiration) with microscopic exposure of the epididymal tubules or PESA (**P**ercutaneous **E**pididymal **S**perm **A**spiration) from directly epididymal head.

The equipment needed for PESA is readily available and inexpensive: a 23 gauge butterfly needle, a 10 ml syringe, a small hemostat, and 5 ml of sperm nutrient medium.

After the genitalia are washed and draped in a sterile fashion, a cord block can be performed. The epididymis to be aspirated is held in the surgeon's nondominant hand; the head of the epididymis is held between thumb and forefinger. A 23-gauge butterfly needle attached to the 10 ml syringe previously flushed with just enough sperm nutrient medium to moisten the needle is inserted into the caput along its long axis. The assistant pulls back on the syringe to produce and hold 5 mL of negative pressure. The needle is moved back and forth a few millimeters within the epididymal head while the sides of the epididymis are gently compressed to "encourage" the sperm into the needle. When aspirated fluid is seen in the clear tubing just above the needle hub, the tubing is clamped with the hemostat to hold the fluid in place, and the negative pressure in the syringe is slowly released.

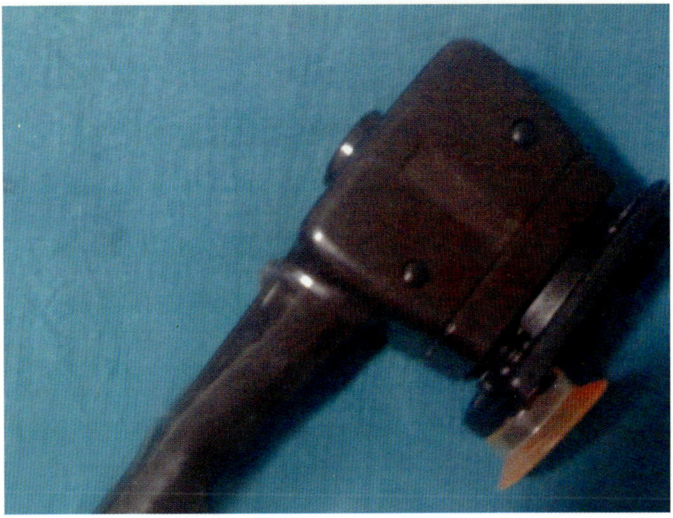

Figure 15.7: Electroejaculator

ANEJACULATION

Anejaculation can be psychogenic (anorgasmic) or organic (obstructive causes/ neurogenic causes). Treatment includes psychosexual counseling, drugs like ephedrine/vibrator therapy (Fig. 15.7) or electroejaculator.

Vibrator therapy is best suited for situational anejaculation/anorgasmic ejaculation. The vibrator works by providing high intensity stimulus to the penis. The procedure should be carried out in isolated room. The patient should be totally relaxed. He should empty bladder and the vibrator is placed under the frenulum which most sensitive part of penile anatomy. The vibrations are continued till ejaculation occurs (usually up to 30 minutes) but sometimes up to 2 hours. Some patients may need 2 or 3 sessions before they ejaculate.

ELECTROEJACULATOR

If vibrator therapy fails and in patients of spinal cord injury electroejaculation is necessary. The electroejaculator stimulates the pelvic nerves and results in ejaculation. It should be done in general anesthesia (Except for spinal cord injury patients).

In patients having retrograde ejaculation; before vibrator stimulation and electroejaculator alkalinizer should be given to provide alkaline medium for the sperms released in bladder urine. After the retrograde ejaculation the urine should be collected with catheterization after using coconut oil as lubricant.

So for the male infertility clinic, armamentarium like penile vibrator, Prader's orchidometer, facility for semen analysis, hand held Doppler for varicocele evaluation and a surgical microscope with good resolution and magnification. The andrological set-up will be definitely more complete if electroejaculator is available although its cost may prevent many clinicians not to go for it.

16 Understanding Sexual Dysfunction: An Overview

DEFINITION

Sexual dysfunction is broadly defined as the inability to fully enjoy sexual intercourse.

REVISED CLASSIFICATION DSM-5

There are now only three female dysfunctions and four male dysfunctions in DSM-5, as opposed to five and six, respectively, in the DSM-IV.

REVISED DIAGNOSTIC CRITERIA APPLICABLE TO ALL DIAGNOSES (TABLE 16.1)

- DSM-5 sexual dysfunction diagnoses now require a minimum **duration** of **6 months** as well as a **frequency** of **75–100%**
- The disorder must be deemed to have caused **significant distress**
- In addition to the existing specifiers of lifelong vs acquired and generalized vs situational, a **new severity scale** was added: the disorder can be described as **mild, moderate or severe**.

A new group of criteria called "associated features" was introduced. It is subdivided into 5 categories: (1) partner factors (e.g. partner sexual problem; partner health status); (2) relationship factors (e.g. poor communication, discrepancies in desire for sexual activity); (3) individual vulnerability factors (e.g. poor body image; history of sexual or emotional abuse), psychiatric comorbidity (e.g. depression; anxiety), or stressors (e.g. job loss; bereavement); (4) cultural or religious factors (e.g. inhibitions related to prohibitions against sexual activity or pleasure; attitudes toward sexuality); and (5) medical factors relevant to prognosis, course, or treatment.

Table 16.1: Revised diagnostic criteria applicable to all diagnoses

DSM-IV-TR Diagnoses	*Changes in DSM-5*
Female dysfunctions:	
Female hypoactive desire disorder	Merged into:
Female arousal disorder	**Female sexual interest/arousal disorder**
Female orgasmic disorder	Unchanged
Dyspareunia	Merged into:
Vaginismus	**Genitopelvic pain/penetration disorder**
Male dysfunctions:	
Male erectile disorder	*Changed to* **Erectile disorder**
Hypoactive sexual desire disorder	*Changed to* **Male** hypoactive sexual desire disorder
Premature ejaculation	*Unchanged*
Male orgasmic disorder	*Changed to* **Delayed ejaculation**
Male dyspareunia	
Male sexual pain	*Deleted*
Other dysfunctions:	
Sexual aversion disorder	*Deleted*
SD due to a general medical condition	
Substance/medication-induced sexual dysfunction	*Unchanged*
Sexual dysfunction NOS	*Replaced by* **Other specified sexual dysfunctions** *and* **Unspecified sexual dysfunction**

Note. Individual changes to DSM nomenclature and criteria are in bold

TRADITIONAL FEMALE SEXUAL RESPONSE CYCLE (FIG. 16.1)

Two models of the sex response cycle have received attention in the literature.[1,2] Masters and Johnson were among the early researchers to scientifically study the human sexual response cycle from a physiological standpoint.[1] They postulated that the sexual response cycle consisted of four successive phases: excitement, plateau, orgasm, and resolution.

In 1979, Kaplan[2] proposed adding the aspect of desire as shown here.[1] This model is somewhat simplistic and does not factor in the more complex emotions involved in a woman's sexual response:

- Blood accumulates in the pelvic area
- Vaginal lubrication begins

- The vagina expands and lengthens
- Labia, clitoris, and sometimes the breasts enlarge
- Labia enlarge more and labia minora darken
- Respiration and heart rate increase
- Vaginal introitus narrows
- Respiration and heart rate decrease to normal
- Labia, clitoris return to normal states
- Occasional soreness in clitoral region.

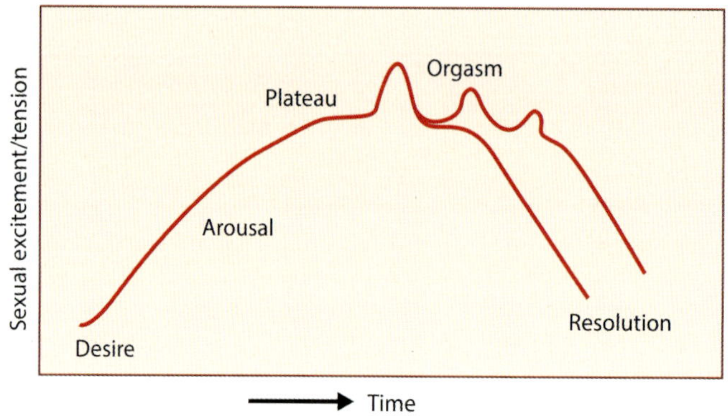

Figure 16.1: Traditional model of female sexual response cycle[1,2]

PROPOSED INTIMACY-BASED FEMALE SEX RESPONSE CYCLE (FIG. 16.2)

Women's sexual arousal is complex and encompasses numerous biopsychosocial aspects.

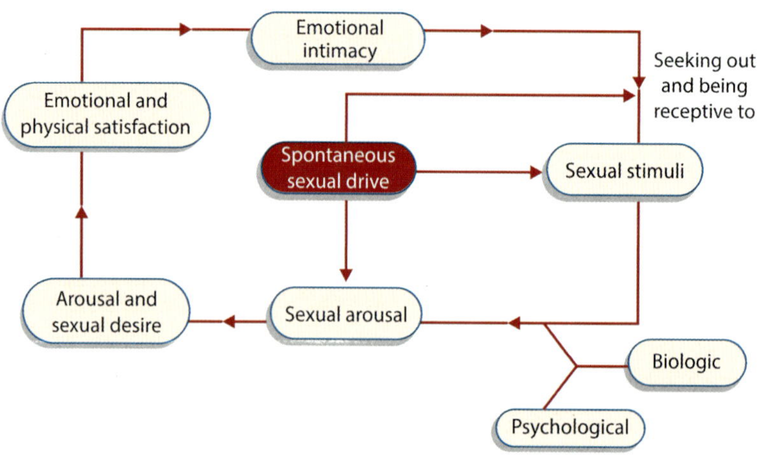

Figure 16.2: Proposed intimacy-based female sex response cycle (circular model) (*Source:* Basson R. Med Aspects Hum Sex. 2001;1:41-2)

In the past 50 years the sexual response has been studied and documented. Knowing the normal response helps to understand how to help dysfunctional couples.

- **Diagnostic and Statistical Manual of Mental Disorders DSM-5 2013**
  - Female sexual interest/arousal disorder
  - Absent/reduced interest/arousal related to sexual activities, thoughts, fantasies, etc.
  - Absence of (1) initiation of sexual activity, (2) excitement and pleasure, (3) response to sexual cues and sensation genital or non-genital.
  - Becomes persistent problem for relationships
  - Lifelong vs. acquired; generalized vs. situational; mild, moderate or severe
  - Female orgasmic disorder
    - 75–100% absence
    - Delay, infrequency or absence of orgasm and/or reduced intensity of orgasm sensations lasting more than 6 months
    - Reduced intensity of orgasm
    - Wide estimates of prevalence: 10–42%
    - 15% of women do not report experience of orgasm
    - Lifelong vs. acquired; generalized vs. situational, also never; mild, moderate or severe
  - Genitopelvic pain/penetration disorder
    - Difficulties with, (a) vaginal penetration during intercourse, (b) pain during penetration, (c) fear or anxiety about pain of penetration during or after sex, (d) contraction of pelvic floor muscles during sex
    - Lasting more than 6 months
    - 15% of women report some pain during intercourse
    - Lifelong vs. acquired; mild, moderate or severe
- **Diagnostic and Statistical Manual of Mental Disorders DSM**
  - Sexual pain disorders (Figs 16.3A and B).

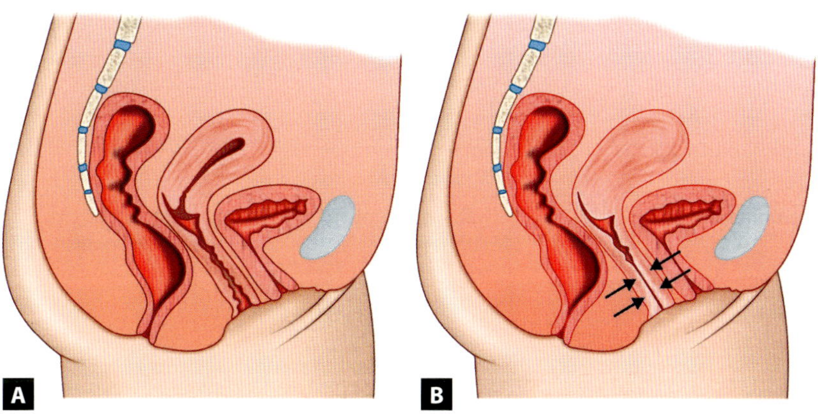

Figures 16.3A and B: Genito-pelvic pain/penetration disorder (A) Dyspareunia; (B) Vaginismus

Female Sexual Dysfunction Risk Factors

Hypertension, smoking and substance abuse, hyperlipidemia, previous pelvic surgery and past psychological trauma.

Several pharmacotherapies can increase the risk of female sexual dysfunction: Several pharmacotherapies may result in sexual side effects. For example, the SSRIs have been associated with delayed or absent orgasm, depending on the balance between serotonergic, noradrenergic, and dopaminergic activity and dose. Patients should be questioned on the use of these pharmacotherapies as well as use of over-the-counter and alternative medicines during the medical history (Table 16.2).

Certain medical conditions can increase the risk of female sexual dysfunction: A complete medical history should be conducted in order to rule out a female sexual dysfunction (FSD) secondary to an underlying medical condition (Table 16.3). Untreated depression is associated with decreased desire due to alterations in serotonergic activity. Diabetes impairs arousal and orgasm, possible due to uncontrolled hyperglycemia. Thyroid disease is often associated with decreased desire that resolves with treatment. Coronary artery disease or a history of myocardial infarction may negatively impact desire or arousal due to fear of causing another event. Neurologic disease such as multiple sclerosis and spinal cord injuries may impair arousal and orgasm due to injury in brain regions that process sexual stimuli. Androgen insufficiency resulting from oophorectomy may result in hypoactive desire. Estrogen deficiency in postmenopausal women is associated with vaginal atrophy, pain, and impaired arousal. Partner health issues may also contribute to an FSD.

Table 16.2: Drugs causing sexual dysfunction

Antidepressants and mood stabilizers	SSRIs SNRIs Tricyclics Antipsychotics	Benzodiazepines Antiepileptics MOAIs
Antihypertensives	Beta-blockers Alpha-blockers	Diuretics
Cardiovascular agents	Lipid-lowering agents Digoxin	
Hormones	Oral contraceptives Estrogens Progestins	Antiandrogens GnRH agonists
Others	Histamine H_2-receptor blockers Narcotics Amphetamines Anticonvulsants	

Basson R, Schultz WW. Lancet. 2007;369:409-24; Kingsberg SA, Janata JW. Urol Clin North Am. 2007;34:497-506.

Table 16.3: Certain medical conditions can increase the risk of female sexual dysfunction	
Condition	*Effects on sexual function*
Depression	Decreased desire
Diabetes	Impaired arousal and orgasm
Thyroid disease	Decreased desire
Cardiovascular disease	Impaired arousal
Neurologic diseases	Impaired arousal and orgasm
Androgen insufficiency	Decreased desire
Estrogen deficiency	Impaired arousal
Basson R, Schultz WW. Lancet. 2007;369:409-24; Kingsberg SA, Janata JW. Urol Clin North Am. 2007;34:497-506.	

Causes of Female Sexual Dysfunction

In addition to the biological factors that may contribute to FSD, psychological factors also play a significant role. Stress, a history of sexual or substance abuse, and sociocultural influences may have a negative impact on a woman's sexual function.

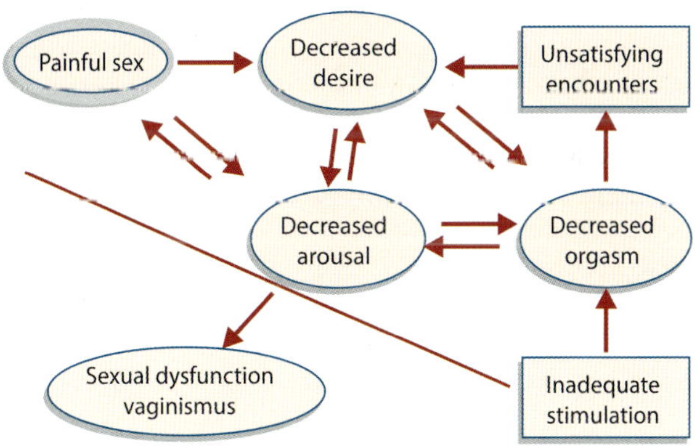

Figure 16.4: Female sexual dysfunction

Organic Causes

- Diabetes, heart disease, neurological disorders, hormonal imbalances
- Chronic disease (liver or renal)
- Arthritis and urinary incontinence
- Substance abuse may have negative effect in arousal
- Pregnancy and postpartum states (prolonged lactation)
- Medication has an influence: On desire, arousal, ability to attain orgasm.

Combination of surgical and psychological effects:

- Gynecological malignancy—74% reported decreased desire and 40% reported dyspareunia.

Surgical effects

- Breast cancer survivors—21-39% incidence of sexual dysfunction
- Hysterectomy for benign disease—30% reported decreased response.

Psychosocial factors can increase the risk of female sexual dysfunction: In addition to the biological factors that may contribute to FSD, psychological factors also play a significant role. Stress, a history of sexual or substance abuse, and sociocultural influences may have a negative impact on a woman's sexual function (Fig. 16.4). Relationship issues can be the cause, effect, or both of FSD which include Sexual boredom, dislike of partner, anger, fear, power differences, control issues, fallen out of love, lack of sexual attraction infidelity, disappointment, perceived selfishness, money, kids, in-laws, different values or interests, abuse, partner's psychological disturbance. Sexual performance concerns—an important issue is the understanding of the male partner, who often feels that, like him, his partner cannot fully enjoy sexual activity without orgasm. Hence, there is an enormous pressure on the woman to achieve orgasm.

Cultural influences/religious taboos and negative upbringing may have instilled the belief that sex is dirty and masturbation is unnatural, and unhealthy education and permission should be given by the therapist to alter such misconception. Partner sexual dysfunction (ED) may cause desire disorder in women. Alcohol and subabuse—Sexuality and partner relationships were found to be more stressful and conflicting among women alcoholics and subabusers. Decrease in desire, impaired arousal, lubrication, delayed orgasm are experienced by alcoholics and subabusers.

Depressive states increases feeling of fatigue thereby diminishing desire for sex causing inhibition of desire and arousal.

Psychological/Psychosocial Causes

- Marital/relationship problems can be the cause and effect or both
- Depression, stress/anxiety
- Cultural influences and religious taboos
- Negative upbringing (feeling of guilt)
- Sexual performance concerns
- Partner sexual dysfunction
- Past sexual, emotional, physical trauma
- Past interpersonal relationships
- Alcohol and substance abuse
- Low self-esteem (poor body image).

Diagnosis/Evaluation

Non-judgemental, direct questions are best use for evaluation. Clinicians should inquire about sexual function in all patients. This screening should be carried out in private, when the patient is fully clothed. Studies indicate that physicians' characteristics, such as level of eye contact, seat positioning, and relaxed nature, have an impact on patients' comfort when discussing sexuality. Clinicians can increase their own level of comfort by practicing sexual terminology.

Complete history and physical examination is critical and should include:

- Pap and pelvic exams
- Attitude towards sex
- Past trauma/sexual abuse
- Relationship problems
- Sexual orientation
- Substance abuse
- Medical history.

Elements of a Routine Medical Assessment for Female Sexual Dysfunction

- Past medical history
- Physical examination
  - Inspection of external genitalia
  - Mono- and bimanual examinations
- Laboratory tests
  - Thyroid function tests
  - Hormone profile
  - Fasting glucose.

Patients should be queried on their past and present medical histories to identify any biological factors that may contribute to female sexual dysfunction. A physical examination, including a urogynecologic examination, should be performed to identify anatomical abnormalities or pathologies that may compromise, mask, or be masked by sexual function.

Comprehensive Sexual Assessment

- Nature of problem
- Duration of problem
- Primary or secondary
- Situational or generalized
- Relationship problems
- Stressors
- Sexual problems in partner
- History of physical, emotional or sexual abuse.

Information obtained from this assessment can be used to identify which domain(s) of sexual response are affected, determine the timeline, dissect the etiology of FSD, and provide information on the most appropriate treatment approach.

BRIEF SCREENING FOR FEMALE SEXUAL DYSFUNCTION

Clinicians should inquire about sexual function in all patients. Assessment should be carried out in private, when the patient is fully clothed. Studies indicate that physicians' characteristics, such as level of eye contact, seat positioning, and relaxed nature, have an impact on patients' comfort when discussing sexuality.

Detailed sexual history that clinician can collect when there is time to do so. Information from the assessment can be used to dissect the etiology of female sexual dysfunction.

- First sexual experience
- Approximate number of partners
- Gender and orientation development
- Sexually transmitted infections
- Pregnancies
- Past history of sexual problems
- Current/past history of physical or sexual abuse (domestic violence to be covered separately but keep in mind)
- Sexual messages received growing up
- Significant sexual experiences—both positive and negative, particularly any abuse (psychological, physical, sexual)
- History of sexual relationship with current partner.

ALGORITHM FOR ESTABLISHING A DIAGNOSIS OF FEMALE SEXUAL DYSFUNCTION

Algorithm for establishing a diagnosis of FSD may be helpful for a brief comparison of all the possible female sexual dysfunctions and their key criteria and can be used for making a diagnosis of sexual dysfunction (Fig. 16.5).

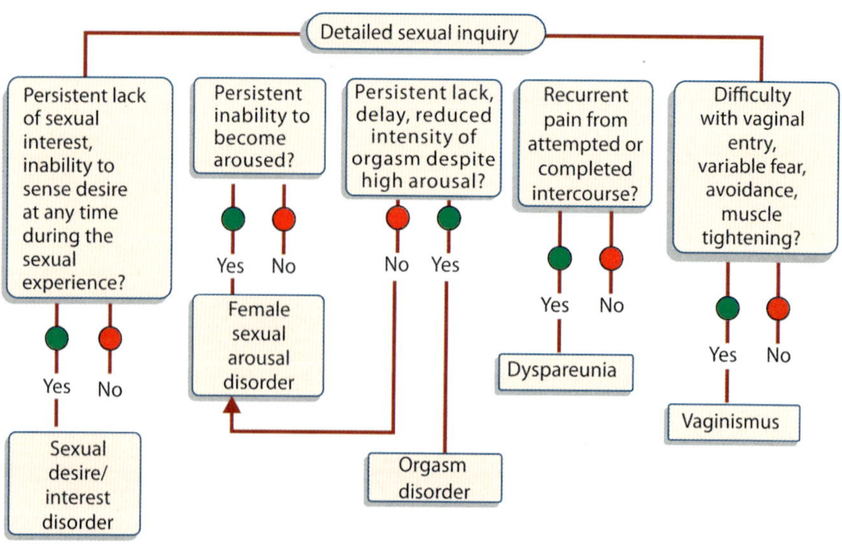

Figure 16.5: Algorithm for establishing a diagnosis of female sexual dysfunction (*Source:* Basson R, et al. J Sex Med. 2004;1:24-34)

GENERAL TREATMENT GUIDELINES

- Education, Education, Education!! (anatomy, sexual function, effects of pregnancy, menopause and aging)
- Enhancing stimulation (erotic materials, encouraging communication during sexual activity, masturbation)
- Distraction techniques (fantasy, Kegel exercises with intercourse, background music or television)
- Encouraging noncoital behaviors (massage, sensate focus exercise)
- Minimize pain (positional, lubricants, warm baths, biofeedback, NSAIDs prior to intercourse)
- Treatment depends on the cause, if organic, appropriate medical/surgical interventions. Plus or minus sex counseling. If psychogenic then psychotherapy/sex therapy/marital therapy/behavior therapy or CBT can be used.
- Lifestyle modification counseling should be included in all cases.

Holistic Approach for Management of Female Sexual Dysfunction (Table 16.4)

Most successful treatments for female sexual dysfunction are "Psychophysiological", in that physiological change circularly interacts with psychological change. In the enthusiasm for new physiologic approaches, there has been a strong tendency to overlook the evidence that does exist for efficacious psychological treatments.

- The numerous psychological factors that motivate a woman to begin her sexual experience must always be kept in the forefront when pharmacotherapy is considered.
- Since a psychological treatment does impact sexual physiology, we need to continue to develop psychological approaches both out of intellectual interest and out of respect for the choices of patients preference.
- The prescription of a physiologic treatment which ignores the fact that human sexuality is infused with individual meaning may invite further interference with sexual functioning.

Treatment of Vaginismus

Figure 16.6 shows treatment of vaginismus.

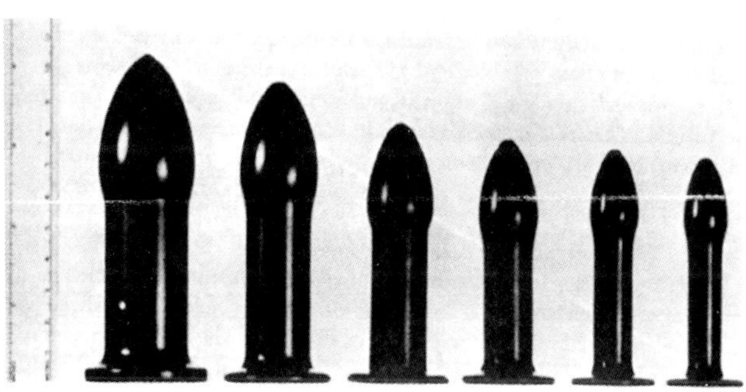

Figure 16.6: Treatment of vaginismus (dilators)

Table 16.4: Psychological approaches to female sexual dysfunction

Disorder	*Psychological approaches*
Hypoactive sexual interest/ desire disorder	• The most common of disorders. Treatment must be individualized to the factors that is inhibiting sexual interest • Some couples require marital therapy prior to focusing directly on enhancing sexual activity. Declining sex is sometimes one of the few areas where someone who feels dominated in most other areas of a marriage may still exert control • Many couples will need to direct focus on the sexual relationship through education and couple assignments they expand the variety and time devoted to sexual activity plus bridge the gap in their sexual expectations • Some couples will also need to focus on how they may sexually approach their partner in more interesting and desirable ways, and how to more gently and tactfully decline a sexual invitation • The psychological portion of treatment is directed at teaching how to focus on pleasurable thoughts and feelings about sex, i.e. sensate focus • Strategies to alleviate anxiety by employing distraction techniques (spectatoring), fantasizing or listening to music are helpful • Treating communication and other relationship issues believed to cause or maintain the disorder
Sexual orgasmic disorder	• Unlike men, in women orgasm is a learned and not an automatic process, 5–15% have never had an orgasm, anorgasmia, usually result of sexual inexperience, performance anxiety or past experiences that have let to inhibition • The goals of such treatment relies on decreasing anxiety; minimizing distraction and inhibition and maximizing stimulation • Methods to minimize inhibition include spectatoring (observing oneself from a third party perspective), fantasizing or listening to music. Stimulation may include masturbation and or use of vibrator as needed • Individual and couple counseling sessions and sex therapy may be effective for treatment of orgasmic disorder. Usually responsive to therapy • Occurs usually due to sexual inexperience or lack of sufficient stimulation
Genito-pelvic pain/ penetration disorder	• Vaginismus—treatment consists of progressive muscle relaxation and vaginal dilation exercises using plastic dilators. It is important that the use of dilators proceeds in a systematic progression under the direction of a professional and should actively involve the woman's sexual partner. The treatment include gradually more intimate contact eventually culminating in successful and pain free intercourse. Sex education about physiology, sexual response cycle and myths about sex is also very important to counter sexual naivety and dispel any misinformation • In cases where there is a strong phobic avoidance component, the use of hypnosis and relaxation may be useful • Dyspareunia—progressive muscle relaxation exercises may help a woman regain control over vaginal muscles, reducing pain and making sexual intercourse more pleasurable in deep dyspareunia • In long-term pain disorder psychotherapy, pain control strategies and systematic desensitization are helpful

REFERRAL FOR FEMALE SEXUAL DYSFUNCTION

Clinicians with a low level of comfort or expertise in treating patients with female sexual dysfunction (FSD) may wish to refer their patient to a specialist to improve outcomes. Patients with complex FSD or accompanying relationship problems may also benefit from specialized treatment. Options for referral include Sexologist, sex therapists or an OB/GYN, primary care practitioner specializing in FSD. Patients should be reminded that referral is a common procedure in order to alleviate any fears or feelings of rejection by their clinician.

BASIC TREATMENT STRATEGIES FOR 'FSD' (TABLE 16.5)

- Estrogen replacement therapy has been shown to correlate positively with sexual activity, enjoyment and desire, although the findings are not universal.
- Testosterone therapy for treatment of disorders of desire.

Table 16.5: Pharmacotherapeutic approaches to female sexual dysfunction

Disorder	*Pharmacotherapeutic approaches*
Hypoactive sexual disorders	• Transdermal testosterone gel (phase 3 trial underway), inhaled sprays and vaginal ring containing testosterone under research • Estrogen therapy may help some.
Sexual arousal disorder	• Vacuum device which increases clitoral and external genitalia blood flow • Local application of a vasodilator is another approach to increase blood flow • Number of centrally acting agents are also under investigation
Orgasmic disorder	• There are no pharmacotherapeutic approaches of treating orgasmic disorder but the vacuum device which increases genitalia blood flow is also approved • EROS therapy
Pain disorder	• Dyspareunia—vaginal lubrication gel and variety of local or systemic hormone therapies can be used (postmenopausal women) • Vaginismus—dilators can be used

Screening

- Baseline testosterone levels (free and total)
- Baseline lipid profile
- Baseline liver enzyme levels
- Mammography
- Papanicolaou smear.

Initiate Therapy

- Combination product (Estratest or Estratest hs)
- Methyltestosterone (Android), 1.25 to 2.5 mg daily

- Micronized oral testosterone, 5 mg twice daily
- Testosterone proprionate 2% in petroleum applied daily to every other day
- Testosterone injectables/pellets.

Re-evaluation at Three to Four Months

- Repeat testosterone levels, lipid profile, liver enzyme levels
- Monitor symptoms, side effects.

Continued Therapy

- Taper to lowest effective dosage
- Monitor lipid levels, liver enzyme levels once or twice yearly
- Routine papanicolaou smear and mammography schedules.

Kegel Exercises

Potential Uses

- Increased pubococcygeal tone
- Improved orgasmic intensity
- Correction of orgasmic urine leakage
- Distraction technique during intercourse
- Improved patient awareness of sexual response.

Teaching Kegel Exercises

- Instructional examination with examiner's finger in vagina
- Initial patient home exercise with patient's finger in vagina
  - Slow count to 10, with movement directed "in and up"
  - Hold for count of 3
  - Slow release to count of 10
  - Repeat 10 to 15 times daily
- Consider vaginal weights, biofeedback clinics.

Maintaining Kegel Exercises

- Advise repetitions during routine activities (standing in line, at stop lights, etc.)
- Schedule follow-up appointments to discuss progress.

Devices/vibrators/ lubricants can be used as a basic treatment

- Estrogen replacement therapy has been shown to correlate positively with sexual activity, enjoyment and desire, although the findings are not universal.
- Testosterone therapy for treatment of disorders.

FEMALE SEXUAL DYSFUNCTION—TREATMENT OPTION ON THE HORIZON

- Androgens
- Prostaglandins

- Nitric oxide delivery systems
- Dopaminergic agonist
- Flibanserin—is a drug produced by *Boehringer Ingelheim*. It is currently being investigated as a drug for women suffering from decreased sexual desire. It is a 5-HT1A *serotonin receptor agonist* and 5-HT2a serotonin receptor antagonist that had initially been developed as an antidepressant.
- Disorders of Desire are an area of great interest and research-neuropeptide oxytocin, which affects sexual motivation in animals, may have a role in treating disorders of this phase
- Apomorphine may be used in treating FSD as it is centrally acting through hypothalamus, and also through peripheral organ response-disorders of desire and arousal
- Drugs useful for reducing pain in sexual pain disorder **(gabapentin)**.

DIAGNOSTIC AND STATISTICAL MANUAL OF MENTAL DISORDERS DSM-5 2013

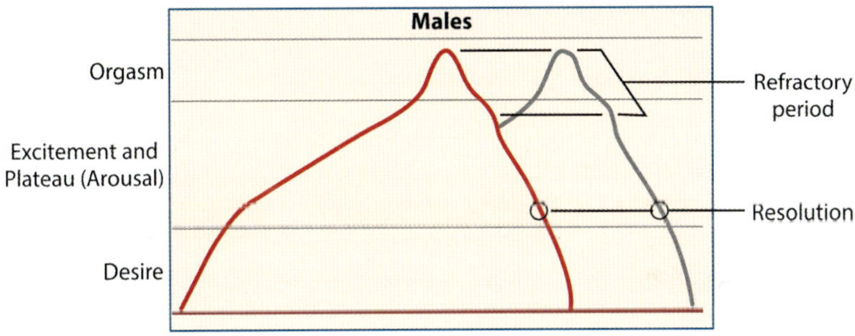

Figure 16.7: Male sexual response cycle

- Figure 16.7 shows male sexual response cycle.
- Erectile disorder
  - Failure to obtain or maintain erection during partnered sexual activities
  - 75–100% requirement
  - Symptom of decreased erectile rigidity
  - More common in men over 50
  - Most problems remit without professional intervention
  - Lifelong vs acquired; generalized vs situational; mild, moderate or severe.
- Male hypoactive sexual desire disorder.
  - Persistent deficient or absent sexual thoughts, fantasies or desires
  - Lasting more than 6 months
  - 6% of younger 18–24 and 41% of older men 66–74 report problems with sexual desire; persistent problem in only 2% of men
  - Lifelong vs acquired; generalized vs situational; mild, moderate or severe.
- Premature ejaculation
  - Persistent or recurrent pattern of ejaculation during partnered sexual activity within 1 minute following penetration or before individual wishes it

- Lasting more than 6 months
- 20–30% of men report cocern about ejaculation speed; 3% have persistent problem
- Lifelong vs. acquired; generalized vs. situational; mild, moderate or severe.

- Delayed ejaculation
  - A marked difficulty or inability to achieve desired ejaculation lasting more than 6 months during partnered sexual activities
  - More common in men over 50
  - Only 75% of men report always ejaculating during sexual activity, >1% report problems lasting more than 6 months
  - Lifelong vs acquired; generalized vs situational; mild, moderate or severe.
- Substance/medication-induced sexual dysfunction
  - Some common causes: (a) alcohol, (b) sedative, hypnotic, or anxiolytic, (c) amphetamine or other stimulant, (d) cocaine
  - Mild 25–50% of sexual encounters, moderate 50–75% or severe 75% or more.
- Other specified sexual dysfunction
- Other unspecified dysfunction

Causal Factors in Sexual Dysfunction

Figure 16.8 shows causal factors in sexual dysfunction.

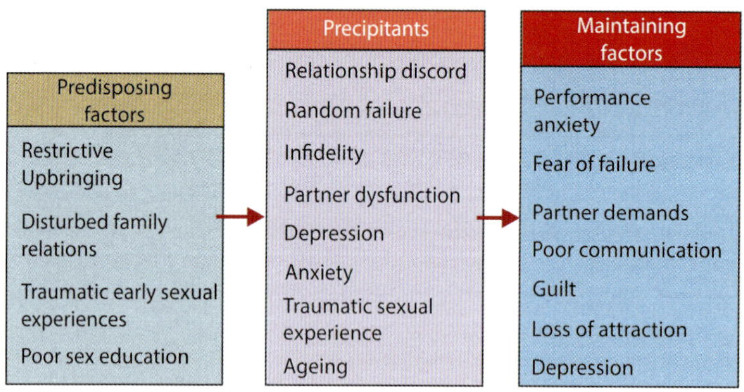

Figure 16.8: Causal factors in sexual dysfunction (Hawton, 1989)

How Common is Sexual Dysfunction?

About 43% of women and about 31% of men have experienced sexual dysfunction based on several surveys. This makes sexual dysfunction one of the most common psychological problem.

SEXUAL DYSFUNCTION ASSESSED IN A SURVEY

- Highest among younger women, with 21% of women aged 18 to 29 reporting physical pain with intercourse. 27% reported experiencing non-pleasurable sex, and 16% reported sexual anxiety.

- Women aged 50 to 59 are one third as likely as younger women to experience pain during sex and half as likely to report non-pleasurable sex and sexual anxiety.

Married men and women report fewer problems with sex than those unmarried. Unmarried women are one and a half times more likely to have trouble climaxing than married women. Unmarried men are more likely to report lack of desire or erection problems than married men.

- Men experience greater difficulty as they age, with men aged 50 to 59 being three and a half times more likely to experience erection problems than the 18 to 29 age group. However, increasing age is not a factor for men who report climaxing too early, anxiety about performance and non-pleasurable sex.

Vicious Cycle of Sexual Dysfunction

Figure 16.9 shows vicious cycle of sexual dysfunction.

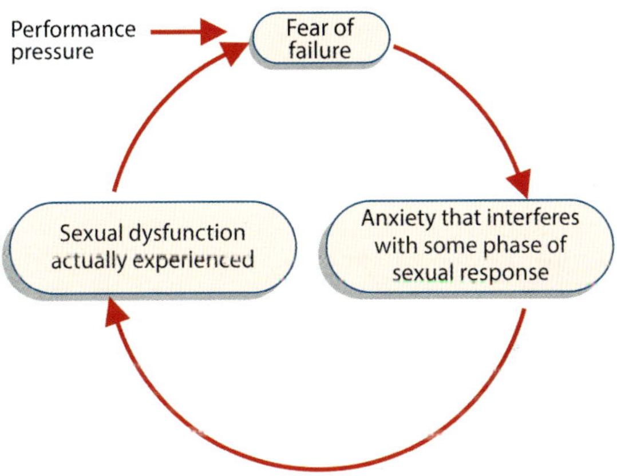

Figure 16.9: Vicious cycle of sexual dysfunction (*Source:* Kelly Sexually Today: The Human Perspective, 6th edn. Copyright © 1998. The McGraw-Hill Companies, Inc. All Rights Reserved.

SPECIFIC TECHNIQUES

- Increase self-understanding
  - Education re-anatomy, physiology, sexual response cycle
  - Instruction on how to masturbate
  - Homework to masturbate in private and later in partner's presence.
- Sensate focus exercises
  - Both partners remove clothes
  - One partner "gives" while the other receives" and gives feedback
  - Initially, no "sexual" touching gradually build up to touching genitals, orgasm and intercourse
  - Gradual reawakening of sexual interest.

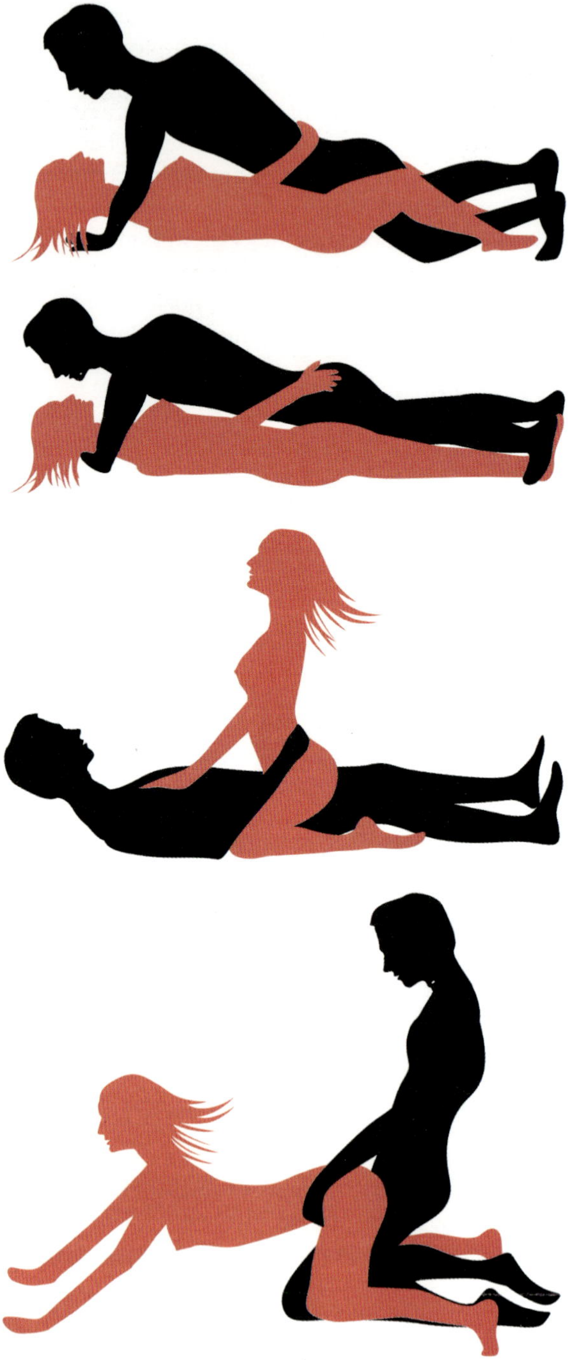

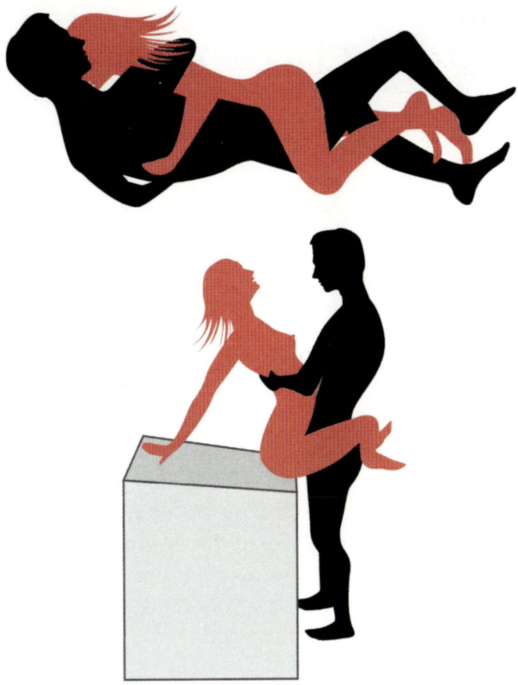

Figure 16.10: Different positioning of sex

- Stop-start technique
  - Manually stimulate penis until close to orgasm
  - Stop stimulation until calmer
  - Repeat
  - May be done by a partner or by masturbation
- Change position (Fig. 16.10)
- Communication
  - Why is it hard to talk about sex?
  - People sometimes lack the specific language
  - Use of "I" statements instead of speaking abstractly.

CONCLUSION

The changes introduced by the DSM-5 aims at increasing its validity and clinical usefulness. It could be argued that, to a certain extent, the fifth edition was successful in reflecting the current state of research in the field sexual disorders.

REFERENCES

1. Masters EH, et al. Human Sexual Response, Boston, Mass: Little Brown and Co: 1966.
2. Kalpan HS. Disorders of Sexual Desire and Other New Concepts and Techniques in Sex Therapy, New York, NY, Brunner/Mazel publications, 1979.

17 Psychosexual Dysfunction: An Overview

DEFINITION

A disturbance of sexual functioning, such as impotence, premature ejaculation, or anorgasmy, that may be caused by one's mental and emotional difficulties concerning sexuality rather than physical disorders.

In psychosexual dysfunction physical problems have been ruled out. Mental or emotional problems are at the center of the dysfunction.

CAUSES

Psychosexual dysfunction is a sexual dysfunction that is due to psychological causes rather than physical problems, medical illnesses, or the side effects of medication (Fig. 17.1).

Some of the psychological conditions include:

- Stress or anxiety from work or family responsibilities
- Concern about sexual performance

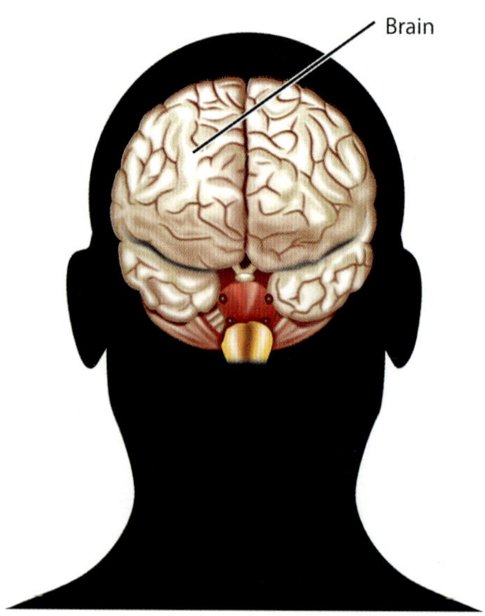

Figure 17.1: Emotional agitation plays major role in sexual dysfunction

- Conflicts in the relationship with your partner
- Depression/anxiety
- Unresolved sexual orientation issues, guilty feelings
- Previous traumatic sexual or physical experience (abuse, rape)
- Body image and self-esteem problems
- Worry or fear about sexually transmitted diseases

Interpersonal relationship causes may include:

- Partner performance and technique
- Lack of a partner
- Relationship quality and conflict
- Lack of privacy

Sociocultural influence causes may include:

- Inadequate education
- Conflict with religious, personal, or family values
- Societal taboos.

RISK FACTORS

Reduced sexual desire or activity is very common among men. Often, the condition is treatable, but first it is necessary to determine whether the dysfunction is caused by physical causes (such as diabetes, heart disease, alcoholism, heavy smoking, side effects of medications (a very common cause of decreased libido or desire), or hormonal problems or psychological causes. Only sexual dysfunction due to psychological factors is called psychosexual dysfunction.

- A risk factor is something that increases your chances of getting a disease or condition.

The following factors increase the chances of developing psychosexual dysfunction:

- Stress or anxiety from work or social situations
- Depression
- Uncertainty about your sexual orientation
- Worry about how you are able to perform sexually
- Fear due to previous disturbing or painful sexual experiences or encounters
- Conflict with the spouse or in-laws issues

Religious, Social, or Cultural Restrictions

- Guilt
- Financial worries
- Family problems
- Abusive relationship with partner
- Negative body image.

Symptoms

Symptoms of psychosexual disorder may differ for men and women.

Symptoms for men include:

- Not able to keep an erection
- Ejaculations are premature (occur too soon)
- Ejaculations do not occur
- Not able to become aroused when appropriately stimulated
- Not able to achieve orgasm
- Inhibited sexual desire.

Diagnosis

The doctor will ask about the symptoms, medical history, and sexual history. The doctor will also perform a physical exam. The doctor to ensure asking about all the medications that are currently being taken. Questions about the partner should also be asked.

Tests may include the following:

- Blood tests to check for problems in your hormones or blood vessels (arteries and veins).
- Test testosterone level: Testosterone is the hormone that creates sexual desire in both men and women.
- Depression scale to measure depression.
- Mini mental state examination (MMSE).
- A test to gauge mental awareness and judgment (also known as cognitive functioning).
- Additional tests for men:
  Snap gauge—A gadget used by physicians to help distinguish if the difficulty maintaining or achieving an erection is due to a physical condition or psychological reasons. Patient wears the Snap-Gauge for two nights in a row to determine if you experienced erections during your sleep—most healthy men experience several erections in their sleep each night.
- Vascular assessment— The doctor needs to make sure the blood flow to the penis is sufficient.

TREATMENT

The most appropriate treatment will depend on the cause of the psychosexual dysfunction.

Some medications can alleviate the symptoms (for example, medications to alleviate erectile dysfunction). However, to successfully manage psychosexual dysfunction, it is important to treat and manage the mental and emotional issues that underlie the problem.

Treatment options for psychosexual dysfunction including in the Flow chart 17.1:

- *Medication:* Medications may be prescribed to treat the symptoms:
  For premature ejaculation: Medications in the SSRI family, such as paroxetine, depoxetine have been shown effective. They may be used on a daily basis, or several hours prior to intercourse.

Flow chart 17.1: Management of premature ejaculation (PE)

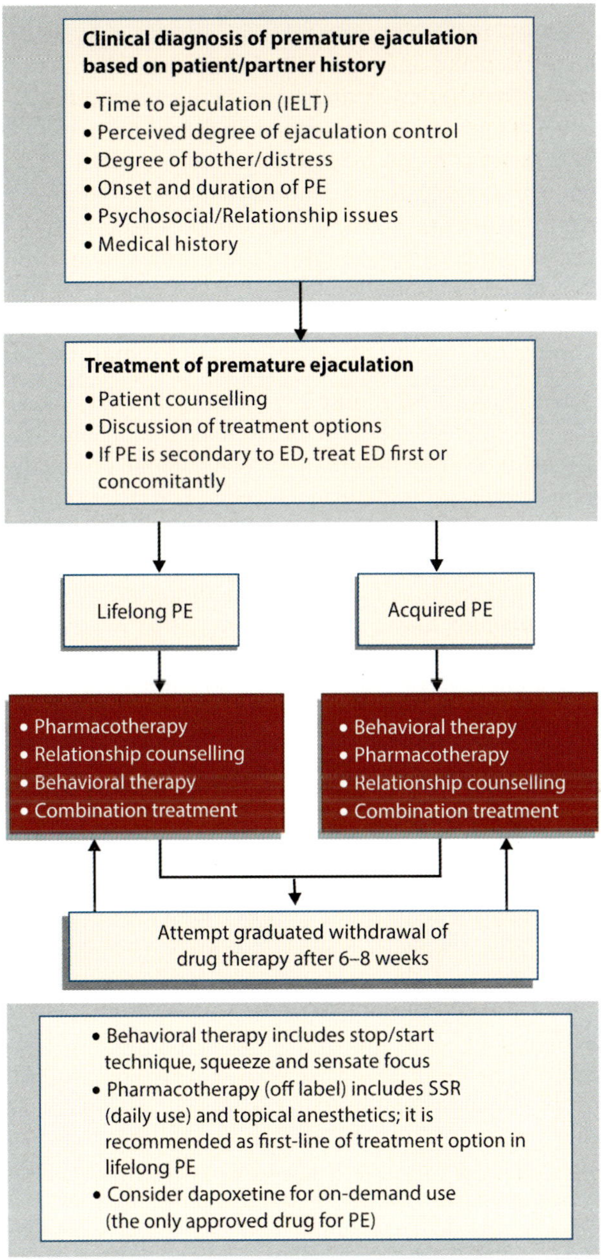

Anesthetic creams may be useful and usage of double condoms may reduce sensations thereby prolonging ejaculation.

- *Psychotherapy:* Patient talks and works with a psychiatrist, sexologist, urologist, psychologist, to figure out ways to deal with stressful or painful issues.
- *Sex therapy:* Sex therapists assist you by encouraging communications, teaching you about sexual fantasies, and helping you focus on sexual stimuli.
- *Behavioral therapy:* A psychiatrist, psychologist, social worker or licensed counselor works with patients to unlearn automatic behaviors.
- *Marriage or relationship counseling:* Couples meet with a psychologist, sexologist or other type of mental health professional to discuss issues, including communications problems.

Some Psychological Treatment Techniques of Premature Ejaculation

Premature ejaculation is sometimes a symptom of anxiety. The amelioration of anxiety by such techniques as relaxation, desensitization, and assertive training has therefore proved helpful in certain instances. Some essentially simple tricks may occasionally meet with gratifying success. For instance, some individuals have managed to delay orgasm and ejaculation merely by dwelling on nonerotic thoughts and images while engaged in sexual intercourse. Others have found it more effective to indulge in self-inflicted pain during coitus (e.g., pinching one's leg, biting one's tongue). Masters and Johnson (1970), however, are not in favor of distraction techniques. The reduction of tactile stimulation (e.g., by wearing one or more condoms, or by applying anesthetic ointments to the glans penis) is also often recommended. All of the foregoing procedures are of limited value (Lazarus, 1978).

- Two very effective techniques for the treatment of premature ejaculation are *the pause* (Semans, 1956) and *the squeeze* (Masters and Johnson, 1970) procedures. The pause technique consists of the female stimulating the male manually until he feels the physical sensations immediately preceding orgasm. At this point, the wife stops stimulating him until the sensations subside, then begins stimulating the penis again, and stops just before ejaculation. As this procedure is repeated, the male begins to develop ejaculatory control. The next step consists of repeating the procedure with the penis lubricated, so that the intravaginal environment is more closely approximated.
- Masters and Johnson (1970) have developed a modification of this procedure in which the wife manually stimulates the penis until it becomes erect. She then squeezes the penis at the coronal ridge for three to four seconds, which causes the man to lose the urge to ejaculate and to lose 10–30% of his erection. The wife waits fifteen to thirty seconds, then repeats the procedure. After practicing for a few days, the couple repeats the procedure with intravaginal containment of the penis, but no thrusting, to produce stimulation. The next steps are intra-vaginal containment with slow movement, and then fast movement, using the squeeze as before.

PREVENTION

There are no known ways to prevent psychosexual dysfunction.

To help reduce the chances of developing psychosexual dysfunction:

- Stay aware of the psychological or emotional health.
- Talk to the doctor or mental health provider if you feel the problems surfacing again, you are experiencing excessive stress, or you anticipate a stressful situation in the near future.
- Spend time alone with the partner often, especially nonsexual intimate time, to help maintain the relationship. This will most likely lead to increase sexual interest.
- Continue to communicate openly with the partner about intimacy and sexual issues.

Index

Page numbers followed by *f* refer to figure and *t* refer to table

A

Acid peptic disease 9
Adenosine triphosphate, production of 2
Alcohol and substance abuse 84
Alli's forceps, application of 31*f*
Alprostadil 16
American Medical System 23
Andropause 61
Anejaculation 41, 77
  management of 43
Antidepressants and mood stabilizers 82
Antiestrogens 65
Antioxidants 65
Antisperm antibodies 66
Anxiety 84
Arousal disorder, female 79
Arterial vascular pathology 9
Arthritis and urinary incontinence 83
Artificial erection 31*f*
Artificial insemination donor 47
Artificial reproductive technology 41
Assisted reproductive technique 65
Asthenospermia, management of 42
Azoospermia 46, 59
  management of 47

B

Breast cancer survivors 84

C

Cardiovascular disease 83
Chlamydia 45
Chronic disease 83
Clitoris 80
Clomipramine 67
Colles, fascia of 5
Color-Doppler
  examination 11
  ultrasound 72, 72*f*
Comprehensive sexual assessment 85
Continued therapy 90
Corona glandis 5
Coronary artery disease 82
Corpora cavernosa penis 5, 6
Corporal fibrosis-post-trauma 9
Corpus cavernosum
  penis 36
  urethrae 5
Corpus spongiosum 5

D

Delayed ejaculation 92
Delayed puberty, management of 66
Depression 84
Desire disorder 88
Diabetes 83
Diastolic arterial velocity 73
Dilated pampiniform plexus 44*f*
Drug therapy 13
Dupuytren's contracture 29
Dysfunctions 79
  female 79
  male 79
Dyspareunia 79, 81

E

Ejaculation 4
Ejaculatory duct 59
  obstruction 50
  transurethral resection of 48, 50
Electroejaculator 77, 77*f*
Epididymal sperm aspiration 47, 52
Epididymis 1, 3, 4, 59
Erectile apparatus 4
Erectile disorder 79, 91
Erectile dysfunction 8, 9, 19, 23, 63
Erectile function, International index of 9
Erection 7
Estrogen deficiency 83
External genitalia, inspection of 85

F

Fasting glucose 85
Female sexual dysfunction
  causes of 83
  diagnosis of 86*f*
  management of 87
Female sexual response cycle, traditional model of 79, 80*f*
Filarial epididymo-orchitis, chronic 66
Fine needle aspiration 52
Fluoxetine 67
Focal spermatogenesis 48
Follicle-stimulating hormone 2
Fungal dermatitis chronic 65

G

Gabapentin 91
Genitopelvic pain 79, 81, 81*f*, 88
Glans penis 5
Goldstein technique 52*f*, 58*f*
Gonadotropin-releasing hormone, release of 2

H

Handheld Doppler 75*f*
Heart disease 9, 83
Hegars dilators 25
Hematological disorders 34
Hormonal imbalances 83
Hyperlipidemia 82
Hypertension 82
Hyperviscosity syndrome 69
Hypoactive desire disorder, female 79
Hypoactive sexual desire disorder 79, 91
Hypoactive sexual disorders 89
Hypoactive sexual interest 88
Hypogonadotropic hypogonadism, management of 66

I

Idiopathic oligospermia 65
In vitro fertilization 59
Infertility 41, 59, 74
Inflatable implant, description of 24
Intracavernosal injection 16
Intracytoplasmic sperm injection 59
Intralesional steroids 65
Intralesional therapy 65
Intralesional verapamil 65

K

Kartagener's syndrome 2
Kegel exercises 90
Keith needle 25
Klinefelter's syndrome 43

L

Labia 80
Local anesthesia 67
Low sperm count 60

M

Mammography 89
Massachusetts male aging study 61
Maximum plasma concentration 64
Medication induced sexual dysfunction 79, 92
Mental disorders DSM 81, 91
Methyltestosterone 89
Müller Helicine arteries 6
Multiple tunica albuginea plication procedure 32
Mycoplasma 45

N

Neurological disorders 83
Nitric oxide delivery systems 91
No needle non scalpel vasectomy 56
Nocturnal penile tumescence tests 10
Non-obstructive azoospermia 52
No-scalpel method 55

O

Obstructive azoospermia 52
Oligo/astheno/teratospermia 41
Oligospermia 65
Open-ended vasectomy 56
Organic erectile dysfunction 10
Orgasmic disorder 89
  female 79, 81
  male 79

P

Pacinian bodies 7
Pain disorder 89
Papanicolaou smear 89
Papaverine 16, 64
Paroxetine 67

Penetration disorder 79, 81, 81*f*, 88
Penile arteriography 12
Penile curvatures 9
Penile fracture 36, 36*f*, 37
Penile implant
 advantages with 24
 complications of 25
 procedure 24
 surgery 26f
Penile prosthesis, types of 23
Penile tumescence rigidity test 73*f*
Penis 4
 arterial supply of 6
 root of 5
 septum of 5
 structure of 6
 transverse section of 5, 6*f*
Percutaneous aspiration 52
Percutaneous epididymal sperm aspiration 52
Peyronie's disease 9, 29, 30
 drug therapy for 64
Phosphodiesterase inhibitors 13, 63
Pituitary luteinizing hormone 2
Post-ejaculate urine examination 48
Postvasectomy pain syndrome 57
Prader's orchidometer 77
Premature ejaculation 38-40, 79, 91, 98
 drugs therapy in 67
 management of 99
 techniques of 100
Prepubertal hypogonadotropic hypo gonadism, management of 66
Prostate 1
Psychosexual dysfunction 96
Psychotherapy 13, 100
Pudendal artery stenosis 12*f*

R

Reproductive system, male 1, 1*f*
Robotic vasectomy reversal 60
Rolling sign 37

S

Scrotal Doppler ultrasound 44*f*
Semen culture 42
Seminal infections 66
Seminal vesicles 1
 transutricular fenestration of 51*f*
Seminal vesicular dilatation 51*f*
Seminal vesicular visualization 75*f*
Seminal vesiculoscopy 50, 51
Seminiferous tubules 4
Sensate focus exercises 93
Sertoli cell 4
 only syndrome 48
Sertraline 67
Sex different positioning of 95*f*
Sex therapy 100
Sexual abuse 85
Sexual arousal disorder 89
Sexual aversion disorder 79
Sexual dysfunction 78, 79, 82, 82*t*, 83*f*, 83*t*, 84-86, 88*t*, 89, 89*t*, 92, 92*f*, 96*f*
 vicious cycle of 93, 93*f*
Sexual interest, female 79
Sexual orgasmic disorder 88
Sexual orientation 85
Sexual pain 79
 disorders 81
Sexual performance concerns 84
Sexual problems in partner 85
Sexual response cycle, male 91*f*
Sperm anatomy 1
Sperm cell 2*f*
Sperm extraction, modalities of 52
Sperm granuloma 57
Sperm retrieval 76
Sperm vitalizers 65
Staphylococcus epidermidis 25
Stop-start technique 95
Stress 84
Surgery 23, 30

T

Teaching Kegel exercises 90
Testes 1, 3
Testicular anatomy 3
Testicular biopsy 48
Testicular sperm
 aspiration 47*t*
 retrieval 52
Testosterone replacement
 therapy for androgenization 66
 types of 68
Testosterone therapy 68
Thyroid disease 83
Thyroid function tests 85
Trabeculae 6
Transrectal ultrasonography 48, 50
Tubal ligation 57
Tunica albuginea 5, 31, 36

U

Urethra 1

V

Vacuum devices 14
Vacuum erection device 19, 19*f*, 71*f*
Vaginal introitus 80
Vaginismus 79, 81
  treatment of 87, 87*f*
Valsalva maneuvers 43
Varicocele 60
Varicocelectomy 45, 46, 46*t*
Vas clip method 56
Vas deferens 1, 3, 59
  congenital bilateral absence of 48
Vasectomy 50, 54
  reversal procedure 57
Vasoactive drugs, intracavernosal injection of 16, 64
Vasoactive substances, intracorporal injection of 15*f*
Vasoepididymal anastomosis 49
Vasoepididymal junction obstruction 49
Vasography 48

Y

Young's syndrome 2